STUDIES IN IMPERIALISM

Established in the belief that imperialism as a cultural phenomenon had as significant an effect on the dominant as on the subordinate societies, Studies in Imperialism seeks to develop the new socio-cultural approach which has emerged through cross-disciplinary work on popular culture, media studies, art history, the study of education and religion, sports history and children's literature. The cultural emphasis embraces studies of migration and race, while the older political, and constitutional, economic and military concerns will never be far away. It will incorporate comparative work on European and American empire-building, with the chronological focus primarily, though not exclusively, on the nineteenth and twentieth centuries, when these cultural exchanges were most powerfully at work.

STUDIES IN IMPERIALISM

general editor John M. MacKenzie

PROPAGANDA AND EMPIRE
THE MANIPULATION OF BRITISH PUBLIC OPINION, 1880–1960
John M. MacKenzie

IMPERIALISM AND POPULAR CULTURE
ed. John M. MacKenzie

EPHEMERAL VISTAS
THE EXPOSITIONS UNIVERSELLES, GREAT EXHIBITIONS AND WORLD'S FAIRS, 1851–1939
Paul Greenhalgh

'AT DUTY'S CALL'
A STUDY IN OBSOLETE PATRIOTISM
W. J. Reader

IMAGES OF THE ARMY
THE MILITARY IN BRITISH ART, 1815–1914
J. W. M. Hichberger

THE EMPIRE OF NATURE
HUNTING, CONSERVATION AND BRITISH IMPERIALISM
John M. MacKenzie

'BENEFITS BESTOWED'
EDUCATION AND BRITISH IMPERIALISM
ed. J. A. Mangan

IMPERIAL MEDICINE AND INDIGENOUS SOCIETIES
ed. David Arnold

Imperial medicine and indigenous societies

edited by
David Arnold

MANCHESTER
UNIVERSITY PRESS
Manchester and New York

Distributed exclusively in the USA and Canada
by ST. MARTIN'S PRESS

Published by **MANCHESTER UNIVERSITY PRESS**
OXFORD ROAD, MANCHESTER M13 9PL
and ROOM 400, 175 FIFTH AVENUE, NEW YORK, NY 10010, USA

Distributed exclusively in the USA and Canada by
ST. MARTIN'S PRESS, INC.
175 FIFTH AVENUE, NEW YORK, NY 10010, USA

British Library cataloguing in publication data
Arnold, David, *1946–*
Imperial medicine and indigenous societies. — (Studies in imperialism)
1. Developing countries. Medicine, 1800–1950
I. Title II. Series
610'.9172'4

Library of Congress cataloging in publication data
Imperial medicine and indigenous societies.
(Studies in imperialism)
Includes revised versions of papers presented at a conference held by the Society for the Social History of Medicine at the University of Aston on Apr. 19, 1986.
Includes bibliographies and index.
1. Medicine—Europe—Colonies—History. 2. Medicine—History—19th century. 3. Medicine—History—20th century. 4. Diseases—Europe—Colonies—History. 5. Diseases—History—19th century. 6. Diseases—History—20th century. I. Arnold, David (David J.) II. Series: Studies in imperialism (Manchester, Greater Manchester) [DNLM: 1. Developing Countries—history. 2. Disease—history. 3. History of Medicine, 19th Cent. 4. History of Medicine, 20th Cent. 5. Public Health—History. WZ59 134]
R484.I47 1988 362.1'09'034 88-9184

ISBN 0-7190-2495-1 *hardback*

Typeset in Trump Mediaeval by
Koinonia Limited, Manchester

Printed in Great Britain
by Bell & Bain Limited, Glasgow

CONTENTS

GENERAL EDITOR'S FOREWORD

Imperialism was more than a set of economic, political, and military phenomena. It was a complex ideology which had widespread intellectual, cultural, and technical expressions in the era of European world supremacy. The 'Studies in Imperialism' series is designed to explore, primarily but not exclusively, these relatively neglected areas. Volumes are planned on environmental aspects of imperial rule, science, education, sexual opportunity, literature, art and design, among others. But in redressing the balance in favour of such multi-disciplinary and cross-cultural studies it is not intended that the economic, political, and military dimensions should be ignored. The series seeks to demonstrate that these can only be fully understood in their wider cultural context and that imperialism had profound effects on dominant as well as on subordinate societies.

The spread of western medicine has often been seen as an unqualified triumph, an emphatic justification for imperial rule. A Eurocentric historiography has depicted disease as one of the great problems Europeans had to overcome in securing their mastery of the wider world. In the nineteenth century, so this tradition runs, western medicine responded to a series of challenges, for example in the epidemiology of both tropical and temperate regions, and pathology, immunology, and pharmacology all took great leaps forward. Not only did this help to make the world a safer place for Europeans, but the health of indigenous populations improved as benefits overflowed to them from scientific advance.

In recent years it has become apparent that the interaction of imperialism with disease, medical research, and the administration of health policies is considerably more complex. Medicine was itself a primary vehicle for imperial ideas and their application, offering richly suggestive insights into the general character of European expansion. Imperialism highlights the fact that medicine is an ideology as much as a practice. It represents a particular way of viewing the relationships between humans and their environment and among peoples, and it illustrates well the necessity of studying the interdependence of metropole and periphery.

This collection reflects the breadth and interdisciplinary range of current scholarship applied to a variety of imperial experiences in different continents. Common themes and widely applicable modes of analysis emerge: the confrontation between indigenous and western medical systems, the role of medicine in war and resistance, and the nature of approaches to mental health. They demonstrate that the application of medical ideas was as much inhibited by administrative constraints as it was promoted by humanitarian concerns; the vigour of the response varied according to the economic significance and the geographical context of the victims; preventive strategies could accelerate rather that arrest the spread of infection; and the connections between disease and malnutrition and their relationship with the social and environmental conditions influenced by imperial policy were but dimly understood. These essays contribute to a major historiographical revision and offer both a guide to current research and signposts for future investigation.

John M. MacKenzie

ACKNOWLEDGEMENTS

Earlier versions of several of the papers in this collection – those by Waltraud Ernst, David Arnold, Malcolm Nicolson, Maryinez Lyons and Terence Ranger – were presented at the Society for the Social History of Medicine's conference on 'Medicine and Empire', held at the University of Aston on 19 April 1986. The Editor wishes to thank the Society for permitting these papers to be included here and for its general co-operation in the preparation of this volume.

NOTES ON CONTRIBUTORS

David Arnold is Lecturer in the Department of History at the University of Lancaster. He is the author of *Police Power and Colonial Rule: Madras, 1859-1947* (1986) and *Famine* (1988), and has written on peasant politics and colonialism in nineteenth and early twentieth-century India. He is currently working on a history of disease and medicine in British India.

I. J. Catanach is Reader in History at the Department of History, University of Canterbury, Christchurch, New Zealand. He is the author of *Rural Credit in Western India: Rural Credit and the Co-operative Movement in the Bombay Presidency, 1875-1930* (1970) and of several articles on Indian peasant history. He is in the course of completing a book on the plague in India.

Waltraud Ernst is currently Research Fellow at the Wellcome Institute for the History of Medicine in London, having graduated from Konstanz University in international politics and psychology. She received her doctorate from the School of Oriental and African Studies in London in 1987, and is writing a book on the history of European insanity in colonial India.

John Farley is Professor of Biology and Adjunct Professor of History at Dalhousie University, Halifax, Canada, and is a parasitologist by training. He is presently working on a history of tropical medicine with particular emphasis on bilharzia. His publications include *The Spontaneous Generation Controversy from Descartes to Oparin* (1977), and *Gametes and Spores: Ideas about Sexual Reproduction, 1750-1914* (1982).

Reynaldo Ileto is Lecturer in the Department of History, James Cook University of North Queensland, Townsville, Australia, and has worked on several aspects of the modern history of the Philippines, particularly its peasant society. He is the author of *Pasyon and Revolution: Popular Movements in the Philippines, 1840-1910* (1979).

Maryinez Lyons is Honorary Research Fellow in the Department of Tropical Hygiene at the London School of Hygiene and Tropical Medicine. She was recently awarded a PhD by the Department of History, University of California, Los Angeles, for her thesis on 'The Colonial Disease: Sleeping Sickness in the Social History of Northern Zaire, 1903-1930'.

Malcolm Nicolson is Research Fellow at the Wellcome Institute for the History of Medicine, London, and works on the history of modern medicine and science. Recent publications include 'Alexander von Humboldt, Humboldtian science and the origins of the study of vegetation' in *History of Science*, XXV (1987). He is preparing a study of the social context of botany in nineteenth-century New Zealand.

Terence Ranger is Professor of Race Relations at the University of Oxford. He is the author of a number of books and articles on African religion and politics and on colonial popular culture in Africa. He is now working on the agrarian history of modern Matabeleland.

Michael Worboys is Lecturer in History in the Department of Historical and Critical Studies at Sheffield City Polytechnic. His main research interests have been in science (especially the medical sciences) in the British Empire. He is at present studying the impact of the germ theory on British medicine 1880-1914.

CHAPTER ONE

Introduction: disease, medicine and empire

David Arnold

'Historians of Africa', wrote K. David Patterson and Gerald W. Hartwig in their introduction to *Disease in African History* published in 1978, 'have generally neglected the study of past health conditions – as well as the role of disease, health care and medicine in history – despite the obvious importance of the disease burden on the African continent.'[1] That statement (partly through Hartwig and Patterson's own labours) seems significantly less accurate today than a decade ago. The history of disease and medicine in general is not now as neglected as it once was and though much of that scholarly attention has focused on the role and impact of disease and medicine in European and North American societies, the rest of the world has come increasingly under scrutiny as well. Some areas have been more extensively investigated than others: the literature on Africa is now impressively varied and wide-ranging;[2] that on South and Southeast Asia remains relatively impoverished, while the Pacific region and Australasia can boast a rapidly growing literature of its own.[3] Much more, doubtless, can and will be done, but it is at least clear that many historians are now aware of the richness of the medical archive and its value for the study of social, political, and economic history.

Perhaps not surprisingly in view of the novelty of the field, there exists little agreement as to what are the central issues in the history of medicine and disease in the extra-European context. There is certainly no consensus over the approach to be adopted. Much of the existing literature has been frankly exploratory in character, doing little more than identifying episodes or trends that appear to be of wider significance or to represent historical turning points in their own right. As in Europe, some writers have confined themselves to the study of a single epidemic, aiming thereby to expose the conflicts and tensions revealed by a society in crisis;[4] others have framed their enquiry in terms of a 'political economy' of health and disease and sought to relate the incidence of disease and the allocation of health care resources to the political and economic structures of colonial rule.[5] A few, even more ambitiously, have described the global dissemination of disease over the past five centuries.[6] Historical demography is one area of rapidly growing interest, while the emerging discipline of medical anthropology has also begun to open up new historical approaches to the study of disease and medicine in indigenous societies in Africa, Asia, Oceania and the Americas.[7] Given such a diversity of approaches and given, too, the continuing division between those who see the history of medicine as an unfolding story of scientific discovery and declining death rates and those who see medicine in a more interpretive light as a 'cultural artifact' and a 'reflection of a society's total being',[8] it is unlikely that any agreed overall picture will emerge in the near future. It would anyway be rash to assume that any kind of natural or automatic congruence exists between the historical experiences of the geographically, politically and culturally diverse lands that formed the western colonial world in recent centuries.

But while this volume cannot lay claim to any such comprehensiveness or universality, it does at least suggest the importance of certain emerging themes and issues in the history of medicine and disease and their role within the context of the colonial encounter. By focusing upon the nineteenth and twentieth centuries, a time of momentous change in the history of western medicine as in the lives of most non-European peoples, by identifying disease and medicine as a site of contact, conflict and possible eventual convergence between western rulers and indigenous peoples, by illustrating the contradictions and rivalries within the imperial order itself, by identifying the importance of medicine and disease to the ideological and political framework of empire, and by drawing attention to the role of medical agencies and practices in shaping the impact and identity of colonial regimes, the contributors demonstrate the centrality of disease and medicine to any understanding of imperial rule.

The main concern here is not so much with disease and medicine as such as with their instrumentality – what they reveal about the nature and preoccupations, the ambitions and the methods of an encompassing imperialism. At the same time the authors do not see western medical ideas and institutions as operating in a cultural void or as structures that could be imposed willy-nilly on compliant indigenous societies. Rather they see medicine and disease as describing a relationship of power and authority between rulers and ruled and between colonialism's constituent parts. These relationships are neither static nor necessarily uncontested: they are subject to influences emanating from the West (not least through developments in medical science during the period) as well as changes arising from within the territories themselves. This complex and shifting relationship is at the core of the case studies that follow, and it is hoped that through their examination of disease and medicine they will help to contribute to a fresh appraisal of the nature and consequences of imperialism itself.

Disease

For many nineteenth and early twentieth century European administrators, reformers and physicians the hazards and depredations of disease were an established part of a hostile and as yet untamed tropical environment. Africa, Asia, the Americas, were all seen to have their fatal and incapacitating diseases, and only through the superior knowledge and skill of European medicine was it thought possible to bring them under effective control. In this view European medical intervention represented progress towards a more 'civilised' social and environmental order. Thus Florence Nightingale, no insignificant figure in the history of Britain's colonial medical policies, saw the creation of a public health department for India as part of a mission to 'bring a higher civilisation into India'. Introducing health care to the subcontinent, she believed, was not only itself 'a noble task': it was nothing less than 'creating India anew'.[9] Similarly for the missionary and explorer David Livingstone medicine offered a way to rescue Africa from its suffering state, 'civilise' it, and prepare it for the blessings of Christianity.[10]

Although the negative health consequences of a European presence were sometimes recognised (as in the case of venereal disease), medicine was taken as a prime exemplar of the constructive and beneficial effects of European rule, and thus, to the imperial mind, as one of its most indisputable claims to legitimacy. Hubert Lyautey, the leading exponent of military medicine as an aid to the establishment of French power in Africa, went so far as to proclaim that 'La seule excuse de la colonisation c'est le médecin'.[11] In a speech made in 1926, towards the end of his active career, Lyautey confessed that colonialism had its 'harsh aspects' and was neither 'beyond reproach' nor 'without blemish'. But, he insisted, if there was one thing that 'enobles it and justifies it, it is the action of the doctor'.[12] Historians, too, have sometimes come close to endorsing this judgement. Writing in terms that echo Lyautey, Lewis Gann and Peter Duignan claimed, in discussing falling mortality rates and surging population growth in colonial West Africa, that 'whatever political disadvantages colonialism might possess, from the biological standpoint its record is one of the greatest success stories of modern history'.[13]

But most recent writers have taken a far more critical view, highlighting the disastrous demographic and social consequences of initial European contact and seeing colonialism itself as a major health hazard for indigenous peoples. The 'successes' of western medicine, if apparent at all, are seen to have arrived late in the colonial era or as benefiting only a fraction of the total population.[14] One line of argument has centred on the often devastating effects of epidemic diseases unwittingly introduced by Europeans and unleashed on societies without prior experience of their ravages and with pitifully little immunity against them. Among the most spectacular examples of this were the smallpox, measles and other epidemics which accompanied the Spanish conquests of Mexico and Peru in the early sixteenth century. These 'virgin soil epidemics' are now believed to have done at least as much as Spanish arms and audacity in toppling the Aztec and Inca empires, decimating the indigenous population with infections to which the conquerors themselves were largely immune.[15] This pattern of bacteriological invasion was repeated in many other parts of the non-European world in later centuries – among the Khoikhoi of southern Africa in the eighteenth century, for example, or among the Australian aborigines, the New Zealand Maori and the Pacific islanders in the eighteenth and nineteenth centuries. Half of the aboriginal population around Port Jackson was thought to have perished from smallpox in 1789: in 1875 a measles epidemic killed nearly a third of the indigenous Fijians[16]. In many parts of the globe, therefore, Europeans had, quite literally, a 'fatal impact' on indigenous society. As Charles Darwin put it, 'Wherever the European has trod death seems to pursue the aboriginal. We may look to the wide extent of the Americas, Polynesia, the Cape of Good Hope and Australia, and we find the same result.'[17] So obvious was the association – in the indigenous perception as well as Darwin's – between disease and the whiteman's arrival by sea that Cook Islanders in the 1830s used the phrase 'I am shippy' when they fell prey to a foreign illness.[18] While to historians of the West the period 1300 to 1600 might appear to be the age of greatest epidemiological onslaught,[19] to historians of large parts of Africa, Oceania, and possibly of South and Southeast Asia as well, the eighteenth and nineteenth centuries, the age of European conquest and colonisation, was an era when epidemic mortality reached proportions almost on the scale of the Amerindian deaths in the sixteenth century.[20] Patterson and Hartwig concluded that, with the possible exception of West Africa, 'the unhealthiest period in all African history was undoubtedly between 1890 and 1930'.[21]

Such assertions are, of course, extremely difficult to substantiate. We know as yet too little about the nature and extent of disease (and other causes of mortality) among the inhabitants of the Americas, Black Africa or Polynesia before the Europeans' arrival, even about cholera and smallpox in India before the establishment of British rule, to make such claims with confidence. It is probably a mistake to assume that pre-colonial societies, even those that existed in virtual isolation from the rest of the world, enjoyed an idyllic existence free from endemic disease and the periodic suffering caused by famine, warfare and pestilence.[22] It may be that the spate of epidemics which afflicted many societies following the white man's arrival have assumed significance simply because Europeans were on hand to record them. Many earlier epidemiological and ecological catastrophes may have preceded them without finding their way into any surviving historical account. It seems improbable, for example, that the ancient trading links between India and East Africa had not brought epidemics of smallpox in their wake long before the nineteenth century, or that pilgrimage routes to and from Mecca had not for centuries blazed epidemic trails across North Africa, the Middle East and western Asia.

But, even with that important caveat in mind, it still seems likely that the scale and intensity of European intervention in the period from the late eighteenth to the early twentieth centuries had a massive, and possibly unprecedented, epidemiological and environmental impact on the peoples of Africa, Asia and Oceania. The reasons are worth summarising.

Europeans forged new epidemiological links, either by relaying diseases (like smallpox and measles) long present in Europe or by establishing ties between parts of the world that had previously had few (if any) such connections with each other. The manner in which plague travelled from Hong Kong in 1894 to Bombay in 1896, to Cape Town in 1900 and Nairobi in 1902, and then to West Africa a decade or so later is indicative of the new facility of disease transmission opened up by modern trade, transport and imperial ties: and the pattern was repeated, in even more rapid and devastating form, in the influenza pandemic of 1918–19. As well as the diseases themselves, European trade and transportation helped the spread of disease vectors, the mosquitoes, fleas and lice by which epidemics were communicated.[23] Even where some contact had existed before 1800 along the African and Asian littorals, nineteenth-century European commercial and political penetration and the creation of colonial infrastructures – roads, railways, systems of labour migration, military recruitment and civilian administration – broke through the coastal barriers and destroyed the quarantining effects that distance and slow land transportation had formerly had on the dissemination of imported diseases. The way in which the 1918–19 influenza pandemic spread along these interior lines of contact and communication in Africa – through soldiers and mineworkers, through markets and railway stations – was a striking demonstration of the degree of European commercial and administrative penetration by the end of the First World War.[24]

Some diseases were transmitted directly by Europeans themselves. The spread of syphilis – known to sixteenth and seventeenth-century India as *firangi roga*, the European disease – was closely associated with European sexual contact.[25] White soldiers, along with local auxiliaries, porters and camp-followers, were potent disseminators of disease. Colonial wars of conquest, the crushing of local rebellions, and the military campaigning of two world wars, brought epidemiological disaster to civilian populations as well as creating high rates of disease mortality among the soldiers themselves.[26] Colonial labour recruitment policies also had serious health consequences both for the workers and for the communities from which they were drawn. Crowded and insanitary conditions in mine compounds and on plantations created micro-environments favourable to the spread of disease among the work force, aided by venereal disease contracted through prostitution, by alcoholism and by industrial pollution. The diseases of the mine, the factory and the city were, in turn, carried back by returning migrant workers to their own families and villages.[27]

On an even larger scale, the nature of the colonial economy and the ecological changes brought about (or hastened) under colonialism, could have far-reaching and enduring effects on public health. The expansion of irrigation canals and the construction of railway embankments created favourable habitats for malaria-carrying mosquitoes in India.[28] In East Africa the spread of uncultivated bush in the wake of the rinderpest, smallpox and famine that hit the region in the early colonial period are thought to have been responsible for the rapid dissemination of tsetse-borne sleeping sickness. In John Ford's damning phrase, the advent of colonialism in Africa marked 'an outbreak of biological warfare on a vast scale'.[29]

In time a colonial regime might provide a health care system that went some way towards meeting the needs of the indigenous population, but this might only partly compensate for the health problems which colonial land and labour policies had themselves helped to create.[30]

But critical though the demographic and social impact of disease undoubtedly is, it does not exhaust the importance of the disease factor in the history of European imperialism and of indigenous experience and response. The history of disease is more than just a history of microbes, mortality and medicine. Inevitably 'man clothes his cosmos in a moral cloak',[31] and in every society, present as well as past, disease, especially epidemic disease, takes on a wider social, political, and cultural significance. The current AIDS epidemic is but the latest reminder of an enduring human disposition to read meaning into collective affliction – to attribute blame and find scapegoats, to see the hand of God or the Devil in the otherwise enigmatic distribution of sickness and suffering. As Terence Ranger's essay in this volume reminds us, different sections of society can derive starkly different messages from a single catastrophe. In a colonial situation, where the cultural and political gulf between rulers and ruled was likely to be peculiarly acute, epidemics might variously be seen as a divine judgement on a benighted people or as a colonial malevolence unleashed against a troublesome race. The concurrence of epidemic catastrophe with European conquest deepened the bewilderment and trauma of conquest itself. The greater the white man's immunity, the greater the suspicion that he must be in some way complicit in the indigenes' misery and sickness.[32]

Disease was a potent factor in the European conceptualisation of indigenous society. This was especially so by the close of the nineteenth century when Europeans began to pride themselves on their scientific understanding of disease causation and mocked what they saw as the fatalism, superstition and barbarity of indigenous responses to disease. Le Roy Ladurie writes (in a borrowed phrase) of the 'unification of the globe by disease' in the period after 1300.[33] In a pathogenic sense there is much truth in this; but perceptually, in the imperial age, disease was one of the great dividers. The emergent discipline of 'tropical medicine' gave scientific credence to the idea of a tropical world as a primitive and dangerous environment in contradistinction to an increasingly safe and sanitised temperate world. As Europe began to free itself from its own epidemiological past, it was forgotten that diseases like cholera, malaria, smallpox and plague, though increasingly banished to the tropics, were part of Europe's own recent experience. Disease became part of the wider condemnation of African and Asian 'backwardness' just as medicine became a hallmark of the racial pride and technological assurance that underpinned the 'new imperialism' of the late nineteenth century.

Beneath the language of medical objectivity and the talk of 'sanitary science', European medical attitudes often remained highly subjective, embodying the social and cultural prejudices of the age. For Christian missionaries in Africa disease was tangible proof of a moral and social sickness it was their religious duty to dispel. The readiness with which endemic yaws in Uganda was mistaken for sexually-transmitted syphilis was arguably not just a case of medical misdiagnosis or even a consequence of current research interests in Europe but also a revelation of missionary doctors' presumptions about African promiscuity.[34] Likewise, cholera in India was more than a dreaded disease. It was associated with much that European medical officers and administrators found outlandish and repugnant in Hindu pilgrimage and ritual – so much so that the attack on cholera concealed a barely disguised assault on Hinduism itself.[35]

The association of diseases like smallpox, plague, cholera and malaria with the indigenous population – a development fostered by the growing understanding of disease aetiology and transmission in the late nineteenth century – deepened European suspicions of the indigenous population as a whole and of those servants, subordinates and fellow town-dwellers with whom they lived in epidemiologically close proximity. Science – and the fear of catching 'native' diseases – provided a pretext for withdrawing from closer social contact and for locating European residential areas well away from 'native reservoirs' of disease in the bazaars, townships, slums and coolie lines. In the extreme case of South Africa medically-inspired social segregation hastened the move towards the racial segregation of an incipient apartheid; but it had its counterparts elsewhere, especially in British West Africa around the turn of the century, and for a while racial segregation became 'a general rubric of sanitary administration set by the Imperial government for all [its] tropical colonies'.[86]

Ill-health among indigenous peoples fostered Europeans' growing sense of their innate racial and physical superiority. In the Darwinian age, little regret was felt over indigenes who fell sick or perished at the mere sight of a white man. It was easy to believe in the superiority of the biologically 'fittest'. Debilitating and incapacitating illness like sleeping sickness – the 'negro lethargy' of the West African slave traders – and malaria fostered ideas of weakness, indolence and inferiority, and contributed powerfully to the development of racial stereotyping by Europeans.[37] The converse of this (as Waltraud Ernst's essay reminds us for the British in India) was that those Europeans who fell physically or mentally sick were quickly institutionalised or sent back to Europe before the image of white superiority could become tarnished.

Disease environments and perceptions of disease exercised a critical influence on the very character of the emerging imperial order. In some regions of the world, the epidemic invasions that accompanied the Europeans' arrival helped to clear the white man's path, brushing aside military resistance and emptying lands suited to white farming and settlement. This pattern, set in the Americas in the sixteenth century, was replicated in later centuries, albeit on a smaller scale, in Australia and New Zealand, at the Cape and in the highlands of Kenya. As A. W. Crosby has argued, European expansionism into the 'neo-Europes' of the temperate regions of the globe, was aided by the operation of a 'biological imperialism' which enabled the establishment of European crops, animals and diseases at the expense of native flora, fauna and peoples. On the other hand, European control was likely to be costly and precarious in areas where the disease factor worked in the opposite direction.[38]

Crosby's biological determinism has much to commend it, but it overlooks the Europeans' capacity to devise structures of exploitation and control that would turn even environmentally hostile lands to their own advantage and profit. Although European mortality on the coast of West Africa was so staggeringly high as to earn it the epithet 'the white man's grave', Europe continued to conduct a highly profitable trade in slaves and gold using African traders, chiefs and other local intermediaries to supplement a minimal and transient European presence. In the West Indies, increasingly a disease environment costly of white men's lives (largely because of diseases imported through the slave trade), African slave labour was used to produce the sugar Europe craved, the slaves being either immune to such diseases or considered cheap enough to be expendable in the pursuit of greater profits. In eighteenth-century India, too, although it was conventional wisdom that new arrivals seldom lasted more than two monsoons, there was no question of abandoning valuable trade and possessions because of high European mortality. It should anyway be remembered that before the mid-nineteenth century Europeans were by no means in agreement as to the cause of high mortality in the tropics. Moreover, Europe's own death rates were still extremely high. A man might as easily die of smallpox (or drink) in eighteenth-century London as in Calcutta, but he might have fewer opportunities to 'shake the pagoda tree' and make the fortune that would set him up for life.[39]

The disease factor could be further mediated through the recruitment of local military and administrative auxiliaries. The recruitment of two West Indian regiments in 1794 was one of the ways in which the British countered the recent devastation caused to European armies in the region by yellow fever.[40] Even after western medicine had become more knowledgeable, British and French colonial expansion and control in Africa and Asia continued to rely heavily on indigenous soldiers, supplemented by smaller numbers of 'seasoned' Europeans.[41] And, in similar fashion, the disease burden in African mines or on tropical plantations was largely shifted from whites onto black or brown migrant workers.[42] Disease before 1900 might discourage white settlement and the use of white labour but it was certainly not an insurmountable barrier to European manipulation and control.

Medicine

Much as Crosby presents an argument for biological determinism in the history of European expansion, so Daniel R. Headrick has recently made a case for technological determinism in opening the flood-gates of nineteenth-century empire. He lists medicine among the several 'tools of empire' that enabled or facilitated western penetration and domination of the non-European world and cites quinine prophylaxis as a specific and critical illustration. Whereas for centuries Europeans, whether would-be conquerors, traders, explorers or missionaries, had persistently fallen prey to tropical fevers, the successful use of quinine by Dr William Baikie's Niger expedition of 1854 proved, Headrick argues, that disease need no longer be a barrier to European exploration and control.[43] As Oliver Ransford succinctly puts much the same point, quinine became 'the prime factor in allowing the whiteman's conquest of Black Africa.'[44]

Headrick's rather selective reading of the evidence leaves several considerations out of account. Forty years after the Niger expedition, a large percentage of European traders, missionaries and officials in West Africa were still dying (or becoming seriously ill) from malaria and yellow fever. Although European mortality in tropical Africa began to decline significantly from the 1890s, this appears to have been due more to the sanitary measures that followed Ronald Ross's discovery of the role of mosquitoes in malaria transmission than to quinine prophylaxis.[45] The use of quinine as a prophylactic was by no means as common in the second half of the nineteenth century as Headrick's account would seem to imply, and although Livingstone was an influential advocate of its use, there was no agreement about the dosage required. Quite apart from the difficulties of obtaining supplies adequate in quality as well as quantity, and the dauntingly unpleasant side-effects quinine could have, insufficient or inconsistent dosage could result in attacks of blackwater fever, which killed or incapacitated many Europeans, such as the missionaries around the shores of Lake Nyasa (Malawi) in the 1890s.[46] It would, therefore, be erroneous to over-estimate the importance of medicine in general and quinine in particular as a weapon in the armoury of nineteenth-century empire. Some medical authorities, like L. J. and J. M. Bruce-Chwatt, prefer to date the most significant advances in tropical medicine to the 1940s rather than the 1850s: only then, they claim, on the very eve of the white man's *departure* from Black Africa, was the 'menace of disease and death' at last 'largely dispelled . . . from the European penetration of tropical Africa'.[47]

Nonetheless, Headrick's argument, even if it exaggerates the specific importance of quinine, does direct attention to a major issue: what part did medicine play in the European imperialism of the late nineteenth and early twentieth centuries? Did it facilitate European expansion? Or did it contribute in other ways to the establishment and consolidation of imperial power? Was its influence confined only to the Europeans themselves or did it have a direct impact on the lives and attitudes of their new-found subjects?

In the long history of European expansion medicine was not a factor of consistent moment. Arguably, and it is a point supported by several of the contributions to this volume, western medicine attained its greatest importance in imperial ideology and practice between 1880 and 1930, the period when European empires were at their most expansive and assertive.

In earlier centuries, and especially before 1800, western medicine was far less domineering in its relationship with indigenous societies, and indeed was largely confined to the Europeans themselves. The Dutch and English East India companies, for example, had shipboard and shorebased physicians and surgeons to minister to the needs of their traders, officials, sailors and soldiers. The first hospitals established at places like Cape Town and Batavia (Djakarta) nestled close to the forts whose occupants they were designed to serve. Only rarely did European physicians offer their services to local rulers – as when the English company's William Hamilton treated the Mughal emperor Farruksiyar in 1714–15 – and even then commercial rather than medical objectives were likely to be uppermost.[48]

Before 1800 (in striking contrast with the late nineteenth century) Europeans commonly sought the help of local physicians, partly because so few of their own were available, partly from a conviction that they were likely to be better acquainted with the diseases (and the remedies) of the place. The Spanish in the Americas, despite their general disregard for the indigenous cultures, adopted a number of local medicines, including the use of cinchona ('Peruvian bark') as a febrifuge; and, until the Inquisition intervened, the Portuguese in western India used Brahmin 'panditos', practitioners of Hindu Ayurvedic medicine, as their physicians.[49] The English East India Company encouraged its servants to rely on local rather than expensively imported medicines, arguing in 1622 that 'the Indies hath drugs in far greater plenty and perfection than here'.[50] In an age when folk medicine still thrived in Europe, white settlers overseas often devised their own medicines making use of locally avalable plants and animals.[51]

During the course of the nineteenth century, however, Europe took a radical step away from medical pluralism. A growing conviction of the unique rationality and superior efficacy of western medicine began to possess European doctors and lay men alike. One factor in this was the momentous discovery by Edward Jenner in the 1790s of cowpox vaccination: this was the first clear demonstration that man could master a major disease and it was a European innovation that was rapidly and confidently exported to the non-European world.[52] Important, too, in changing European attitudes was the growing professionalism of doctors trained and qualified by European medical schools, such as Edinburgh, and dispatched in significant numbers to the expanding outposts of empire. Late in the century the status and authority of western medical practitioners was further enhanced by the development of the specialist sciences of modern medicine. Bacteriology, pioneered by Louis Pasteur and Robert Koch between the 1860s and 1880s, was particularly significant in ushering scientific medicine into an age of 'curative confidence'.[53] The creation of the London and Liverpool schools of tropical medicine in 1899 and the introduction of courses in the subject at the universities of Edinburgh, Durham, Aberdeen and Queen's Belfast (along with parallel developments on the continent and in the United States) raised tropical medicine to a pinnacle of importance in an already prestigious profession.[54]

Nor was this new-found confidence and influence restricted to the laboratory, the surgery and the hospital ward. Recourse to state power to enforce sanitary and health measures (as in Victorian Britain) gave the medical profession unprecedented authority in public life and affairs of state, and this was quickly reflected in Europe's overseas possessions too. One of the characteristics of the period of imperial administration between 1880 and 1930 was the spate of laws, proclamations and decrees giving state sanction to health measures of various kinds. The plague epidemics of the late nineteenth and early twentieth centuries provoked some of the most drastic legislative responses; but smallpox, sleeping sickness and malaria also called forth many of the colonial state's most sweeping enactments (even if, in practice, such laws proved singularly difficult to enforce).[55]

As Malcolm Nicolson's account illustrates for the case of New Zealand, where there were few other educated and trained professional men to hand, doctors became all-purpose 'experts', authorities on matters as diverse as 'native affairs' and town planning. They were recruited as military advisers and impromptu diplomats, as geologists and pioneer anthropologists. If David Livingstone represents an early archetype of the medical missionary and explorer in the mid-nineteenth century, Leander Starr Jameson, associate of Cecil Rhodes and leader of the 'Jameson Raid' into the Transvaal in 1895, epitomises the medical man turned adventurer and politician in the high noon of empire half a century later.[56]

Modern medicine forged new and powerful links between the imperial capitals and distant colonial domains. The turn of the century witnessed the emergence of peripatetic medical specialists, men of the eminence of Britain's Ronald Ross and Germany's Robert Koch, who visited colonial territories from West Africa to New Guinea hoping to bring the benefit of their metropolitan expertise to the service of embattled colonial administrations. The special commission appointed by the British government to investigate plague in India in the 1890s (discussed here by Ian Catanach) was one of the first of many such enquiries – into sleeping sickness in Uganda in 1902, for example, or malaria in Nyasaland (Malawi) a decade later.[57] By this date, whole societies (and not just small colonies of European soldiers, traders and settlers) were being brought under western medical scrutiny. Indeed, the purview of tropical medicine was as wide as imperialism itself, reaching even beyond the formal bounds of empire into regions like Central America where the United States' strategic interests in the contruction of the Panama canal led to a massive campaign to eradicate yellow fever between 1905 and 1913.[58]

All this stood in abrupt contrast with less than a century earlier when European medicine had felt itself competent to deal with only that limited range of afflictions – smallpox, leprosy, lunacy – with which Europeans were long acquainted or which they felt were too dangerous to be ignored.[59] Vaccination, as I argue in the Indian context, made smallpox uniquely subject to western medical intervention at a comparatively early date in the history of colonialism. In many territories, even in the second half of the nineteenth century, vaccination and the segregation of lepers and lunatics were among the few 'medical' services provided. Not only could European medicine at the time offer few other solutions: it lacked even a basic knowledge of the state of health among the great majority of the population, and, indeed, colonial administrations recognised no pressing responsibility for their wellbeing.[60]

The causes and consequences of this rapid transition from white man's medicine to public health during the latter decades of the nineteenth and early years of the twentieth centuries are touched upon in several of the essays in this volume and have received some discussion elsewhere as well. But some of the more salient features of this transformation and of its relationship with a burgeoning imperialism might usefully be outlined here.

There were several imperatives behind increasing western medical intervention. One was the growing realisation, which first gained recognition in India during the course of the nineteenth century, that the health of European soldiers and civilians could not be secured through measures directed at their health alone. As Bengal's newly created Sanitary Commissioner observed in 1865: 'Even if we look no further than the protection of the health of the European soldiers, it will be evidently insufficient if we endeavour to improve the condition of our cantonments alone, and ignore the existence of the masses of the native population by which our troops are surrounded.'[61] It followed, therefore, that the protection of European health could only be attained by measures that took western medicine into the 'black towns' and bustees. Military losses to disease were particularly persuasive in forcing the British (and other colonial powers) to take responsibility for indigenous health. With casualties often heavier from disease than from battle, and given the military's importance to the maintenance of imperial control, the health of soldiers (especially white soldiers) was a high priority of the colonial state. But medical investigations, whether into venereal disease, or cholera, or (as John Farley shows) bilharzia, repeatedly demonstrated that the sanitary and medical security of the military could not end at the barrack gates, but had to extend into adjacent urban and rural areas and even to the indigenous population as a whole.

European self-interest was at work in other ways, too. In an age of expanding world-wide trade and communications, Europe was well aware of its own increased vulnerability to 'tropical' diseases. The cholera epidemics that reached Europe from India several times between the 1830s and 1890s were a persistent and worrying reminder: so were occasional importations of yellow fever from West Africa and the West Indies.[62] In order to counter this threat a series of international (in practice European) sanitary conferences were held from 1851 onwards. In addition to seeking to introduce measures to intercept diseases like cholera before they reached Europe, the conferences also put pressure on individual powers to tackle the more serious epidemic diseases in their own colonies. As the 'factory of cholera', British India was subject to repeated international censure, and the advent of plague there in 1896 put further pressure on the British administration.[63] In an era of competitive imperialism persistently high levels of epidemic mortality were seen as a mark of poor colonial management. King Leopold's requests in 1903 and 1906 for international assistance in combating sleeping sickness in the Congo were partly an attempt to improve the highly unfavourable reputation his regime had already acquired.[64]

Capitalism's internal contradiction between the pursuit of labour efficiency (and thus of workers' health) and the pursuit of profit impelled European colonial regimes and the commercial and industrial enterprises that worked under them towards greater involvement in indigenous health care. There were several interlocking considerations here. Ill-health, especially the circulation of epidemic disease, among African and Asian workers, posed a hazard for white employees and their families. High morbidity and mortality rates interfered with the efficiency and profitability of production in mines, plantations and factories, and discouraged further labour recruitment. In areas where agricultural productivity was adversely affected, as in late nineteenth-century India, by recurrent epidemics and famine, state revenues were directly threatened; while in Africa military recruitment for the First World War highlighted (as it had in Britain at the time of the Boer War) the political disadvantages of an undernourished and unhealthy population.[65] Careless, therefore, though early European dominion often was of the health of its subjects, there was a growing appreciation of the practical returns of investing in the health of the workforce. Given the critical importance of indigenous labour to the realisation of wealth from the colonies, *some* degree of medical intervention was clearly in the colonial interest, providing it did not eat too substantially into the profitability of empire and individual enterprise. The development of tropical medicine and the enthusiasm with which it was taken up by Joseph Chamberlain during his term as Britain's Colonial Secretary between 1895 and 1903 was motivated above all by a desire to protect the lives of the growing number of Europeans living and working in the tropics. But, in an age in which the imperial powers were anxious to unlock the mineral and agricultural wealth of their 'undeveloped estates', the health of indigenous labour was too important to be entirely overlooked. Disease, in the parlance of the 1920s and 1930s, was an obstacle to 'development'.[66] But, because of the self-interested reasons for colonial concern, medical intervention was piecemeal and selective, with scant resources concentrated in areas vital to the operation of the colonial economic and adminstrative system. Thus, while the mine compounds, the plantations, the barracks and the main urban centres were favoured, there was a general neglect of the rural population and of the health of women and children. There was an emphasis on epidemic rather than endemic disease, and upon curative rather than preventive medicine.

The value of medicine as an aid to economic imperialism was most fully realised by the emissaries of North American capitalism. Having undertaken an extensive anti-hookworm campaign in the southern

United States as a way of improving labour efficiency and integrating the neglected South more fully into the expanding industrial economy of the North, the Rockefeller Foundation turned its attention overseas at a time when the United States was embarked on its own expansionist drives. In addition to promoting campaigns against hookworm and later against bilharzia and other diseases of the tropics and funding research on tropical medicine in general, the Rockefeller Foundation, under the guidance of Frederick T. Gates, saw medicine as a superior form of propaganda for the benefits of western civilisation and capitalism and as a way of opening up Asia to American commercial and industrial penetration.[67]

But increasing western medical intervention cannot be explained in terms of immediate material self-interest alone. Medicine was a part of the ideology as well as the accountancy of empire. D. Schoute once argued that when the British occupied the Dutch East Indies early in the nineteenth century they replaced the Dutch company's narrowly 'commercial' medical outlook (aimed solely at keeping its European employees alive) with an 'idealist' vision of medicine in the service of the entire population, Indonesian and European alike. As Schoute himself made clear, the practical outcome of these medical initiatives was small, but the idea of a medicine for the people had, he claimed, a lasting influence on the subsequent medical policy of the restored Dutch administration.[68] The case of the Dutch East Indies, like that of smallpox vaccination in India, and of attempts to take western medicine to the indigenous peoples of New Zealand and South Africa at a slightly later date, all point to the way in which medicine was coming to be seen as having a wider utility in the service of empire.[69] Even before the scientific breakthroughs of the late nineteenth century, imperial powers were beginning to use medicine as a demonstration of their benevolent and paternalistic intentions, as a way of winning support from a newly subject population, of balancing out the coercive features of colonial rule, and of establishing a wider imperial hegemony than could be derived from conquest alone. Given the limited military and administrative resources at the disposal of the early colonial regimes, this was a potentially important weapon in the consolidation of imperial rule, though experience sometimes showed that it might have the reverse effect of deepening mistrust of European motives. While many of these early initiatives lost their way, falling victim to administrative neglect or financial stringency, they paved the way for a return in the late nineteenth century to ideas of wholesale medical intervention.

It was not only colonial administrations and imperial powers that saw in medicine a wider utility. With Livingstone as their mentor, late nineteenth-century missionaries in Africa appreciated the unique opportunity medicine offered to establish contact with the indigenous population and hopefully to gain an influence over them. As Bishop Smythies of the Universities Mission to Central Africa testified in 1893:

> there are some mission fields in which only doctors seem to be able to gain any great influence. There is a fantastic hatred to [sic] Christianity, which can only be broken down by sympathy shown for the sufferings of the body. . . together with the power to alleviate them. It seems as if it is only through medical work. . . that an opening to the hearts of these people can be found.[70]

Missionaries were accordingly recruited specifically for their medical training, and hospitals and dispensaries became central elements in missionary strategy. Missionaries identified themselves with western medicine's 'empirical and rational approach' and through it sought to counter the authority of their rivals, the 'witchdoctors'.[71] Medical work brought missionaries some conversions, though not a few of those they tended and cured took the missionaries' medicine without surrendering their own religious beliefs and their theories of disease causation.[72]

Empire

In the closing years of the nineteenth century medicine became a demonstration of the superior political, technical and military power of the West, and hence a celebration of imperialism itself. It gave expression to Europe's faith in its own innate superiority, its mastery over man as well as nature. Medicine registered the imperial determination to reorder the environment and to refashion indigenous societies and economies in the light of its own precepts and priorities.

As imperial economies and administrative systems expanded and sought a more comprehensive hold over the lives and labour of the people, medicine developed as a central agency for the acquisition of knowledge and the extension of control. Medicine was one of the ways in which imperialism sought to 'know' the people and establish its authority over them – through the vast quantities of information about diseases and health that began to be amassed in statistical and scientific form and through the development of medical agencies, themselves often branches of the state structure itself, that began to reach out into the countryside as well as the towns. The process was not everywhere the same. Sometimes it was slow and faltering: it progressed more quickly in some territories and under some colonial powers than others. But it seemed to reach a general crescendo between the 1890s and the First World War with major campaigns against sleeping sickness, plague, cholera, yellow fever and malaria. In many regions this sudden proliferation of medical power was central to the development of a colonial state and often to the development of the colonial economy as well. Campaigns like those against sleeping sickness in the Congo or against cholera in the Philippines were (as Maryinez Lyons and Reynaldo Ileto both demonstrate) massive exercises in state intervention and social manipulation.[73] Medical intervention impinged directly upon the lives of the people, assuming an unprecedented right (in the name of medical science) over the health and over the bodies of its subjects. Whereas in the pre-colonial past health and medical care were matters for individual initiative or at most communal effort, under imperial rule they became part of a wider process of state regulation and centralised control. Rudolph Virchow, the pioneer of cellular pathology, once claimed that politics was 'nothing but medicine on a grand scale'.[74] In the light of the imperialism of the 1890s and 1900s one is tempted to revise that statement and contend that the imperial medicine of the period was nothing less than politics on a mass scale.

The very nature of late nineteenth-century medicine contributed to this far-reaching medical interventionism. Seeing itself as rational, scientific and universalistic, western medicine defined itself in opposition to the presumed irrationality and superstition of indigenous medicine. The customs and beliefs of the people were treated as obstacles to be overcome, obscurantism to be brushed aside by the new scientific age. They had to be replaced, as one writer put it in 1950, by 'genuine knowledge'.[75] Because the bacteriology of Pasteur and Koch understood disease in terms of microbal invasions, which it was the task of medicine to uncover and counter through the use of specific therapeutics, the social, cultural and economic context of disease was largely ignored.[76] Imperial regimes were encouraged to believe that they could resolve their most pressing health problems by tackling them scientifically, and by showing sufficient resolution to carry them through regardless of local opposition and dissent. The medicine of the late nineteenth and early twentieth centuries was thus of a peculiarly confident and determined kind, believing that it was acting in the best interest of the people. It was confidently assumed that there could be self-contained technical solutions to what were in reality complex social, economic and environmental problems.

The involvement of the military in the medical interventionism of the imperial period is one of its most striking and significant features. In part it reflected the prominence of the army in the establishment and maintenance of the imperial regimes in general, as well as the extent to which the health of the military remained one of the prime incentives behind wider medical action. Governments were prepared to commit resources to the protection of the army's health and sanitation to an extent unthinkable for civilian populations. Apart from missionaries, army medical corps were often the sole agencies involved in research into tropical medicine and constituted the only reservoirs of medical expertise that could be called on in an emergency. In some areas – like Morocco under French rule, or the Sudan under the British, the military monopolised the provision of western medical care until after the First World War.[77] But no less significant was the disposition to see (and speak of) medical intervention in military terms: the French, in particular, 'tackled the battle for health as a military operation', setting up mobile army medical teams to combat sleeping sickness, leprosy and malaria in rural Africa,[78] and the Americans and Belgians showed a similar reliance. It was often felt that the military had the resolution (as well as the manpower) that the civilian administration lacked and was less likely to be constricted by red tape and local opposition. But the military was also likely to ride roughshod over civilian dissent. To civilian eyes, the army's medical operations looked little different from its more familiar military role and the governments were perhaps not unwilling for them to be reminded of imperial might in this way. But one of the consequences of this medical and military assertiveness was that it was likely, as in the Philippines, to alienate the people still further rather than eliciting gratitude and obedience.

The role of the army is a reminder, too, of the importance of considering the manner and the means of European intervention. Attention so far has mainly focused on medical ideas and policies to the neglect of the institutions and agencies through which western ideas and practices were actually relayed to the indigenous peoples. The doctor's race, sex and demeanour could matter as much as the therapies he proffered. Physical contact between doctor and patient could be one of the most direct and traumatic aspects of the colonial encounter.[79] Nor should the importance of indigenous agencies be overlooked. To supplement its own limited manpower and to carry out the more menial medical roles of dressers and vaccinators, colonial medicine looked for local recruits. Initially such subordinates were generally despised and subject to the European prejudices of the day. 'Technical knowledge is easily acquired by the African', the head of colonial Kenya's medical service pronounced in 1926 of African medical assistants, 'but a sense of responsibility, pertinacity, honesty and general trustworthiness are woefully lacking'.[80] But once, for reasons of political pressure or administrative necessity, Asians and Africans began to be given specialist training and professional responsibility the earlier visible foreignness of western medicine became diluted, there could be greater freedom of communication between doctor and patient and rather more sensitivity might be shown than formerly to local sentiment and custom. The Africanisation or Indianisation of medical personnel probably facilitated the eventual acceptance and assimilation of what had once been exclusively the white man's medicine.

The medical interventionism of the late nineteenth and early twentieth centuries threw up its own internal conflicts and contradictions. Western medicine was not moving into a therapeutic and cultural void. Western medical measures threatened many deeply-held beliefs, many long-established social practices. Not surprisingly, they were often greeted with wild rumours, profound suspicion, evasion and resistance. There was violence and rioting as homes and property were destroyed, people were searched, and medical suspects were carted off, like convicts, to hospitals, segregation camps and lazarets. The scale and intensity of these reactions, though by no means universal, raised doubts among colonial administrators about the medical efficacy, the political expediency, and the financial desirability of such massive undertakings. In some cases compromise was preferred to confrontation, even if it meant sacrificing medical objectives and allowing indigenous spokesmen and medical practitioners some part in the conduct of public health campaigns.[81] There was, besides, little agreement among the medical specialists themselves as to how major epidemics like sleeping sickness or plague should be brought under control, and these divisions of expert opinion often inhibited the development of effective and consistent disease-control strategies.[82] Again, as Ian Catanach reminds us for India's plague years, civil administrators were often unwilling to abdicate responsibility to medical officers and experts and insisted that the direction of such far-reaching and politically-sensitive matters must remain firmly under administrative control. The more established colonial power became (or the more it fell back upon the support of 'traditional' elites and social groups in the face of mounting nationalist opposition) the more reluctant it was to undertake a wholesale medical interventionism that might undermine an already precarious status quo.

By the 1920s the administrative and technological limits of western medicine were becoming apparent, as the 1918 influenza pandemic served to remind both the colonisers and the colonised. Although the war and the pandemic acted as a stimulus to the expansion of rural public health in some parts of Africa, the onset of the Depression barely a decade later imposed fresh curbs on public health expenditure. The 'heroic' age of medical intervention was over. A number of major epidemic diseases had by that stage either been curbed or, for reasons independent of western medical action, had ceased to be matters of major colonial concern. There was a growing realisation, too, that disease admitted of few easy solutions, and that much of the ill-health of the colonial world was almost intractably bound up with problems of poverty and nutrition.[83] As Michael Worboys shows, the interwar years brought some recognition that deficient nutrition, rather than major epidemic diseases, now stood in the way of colonial 'development'. But since, as Audrey Richards demonstrated in her pioneering study of the Bemba,[84] diet was largely inseparable from culture, this presented an even larger and more problematic site for state intervention. Although there was some shift from curative to preventive medicine, from epidemic disease to endemic ill-health and undernutrition in the inter-war period, the scale of the problem revealed was too great (and too costly in terms of colonial money and manpower) for most colonial administrations to contemplate tackling in any comprehensive way.

Perhaps the final contradiction of western medical intervention lay in its legacy for the unravelling of empire. The position of western medicine during the Afro-Asian struggles for independence was often ambiguous. On the one hand some nationalists looked to a revival of indigenous medicine as part of a rediscovery of their own cultural roots and rejected the West's alien therapeutics. On the other hand, indigenous practitioners of western medicine were often influential members of the nationalist middle class and colonialism was condemned for its stinginess in bestowing the benefits of western medicine.[85] Perhaps this very ambivalence was an indication of the strength of the impact imperial medicine had made upon indigenous societies.

Notes

I am indebted to John MacKenzie and Terence Ranger for their helpful comments on an earlier draft of this introduction. But neither of those good doctors bears responsibility for any ailments that continue to afflict it.

1 K. D. Patterson and G. W. Hartwig, 'The disease factor: an introductory overview', in G. W. Hartwig and K. D. Patterson (eds.), *Disease in African History: An Introduc-*

tory Survey and Case Studies*, Durham, N. C., 1978, p. 3.

2 See K. D. Patterson, 'Disease and medicine in African history: a bibliographical essay', *History in Africa*, I, 1974, pp. 141–8; D. Patterson (comp.), *Infectious Diseases in Twentieth-Century Africa: A Bibliography of their Distribution and Consequences*, Waltham, Mass., 1979; S. Feierman (comp.), *Health and Society in Africa: A Working Bibliography*, Waltham, Mass., 1979; S. Feierman, 'Struggles for control: the social roots of health and healing in modern Africa', *African Studies Review*, 28, 1985, pp. 73-147.

3 R. MacLeod and M. Lewis (eds.), *Disease, Medicine and Empire*, London, forthcoming; N. G. Owen (ed.), *Death and Disease in Southeast Asia: Explorations in Social, Medical and Demographic History*, Singapore, 1987.

4 The 1918 influenza pandemic has been a particularly rewarding example of this approach. See Terence Ranger's chapter and the references cited there; also H. Philips, 'The local state and public health reform in South Africa: Bloemfontein and the consequences of the Spanish 'flu epidemic of 1918', *Journal of Southern African Studies*, 13, 1987, pp. 210-33; G. Rice, 'Christchurch in the 1918 influenza pandemic', *New Zealand Journal of History*, 13, 1979, pp. 109-37.

5 L. Doyal, *The Political Economy of Health*, London, 1979; M. Turshen, *The Political Ecology of Disease in Tanzania*, New Brunswick, 1984.

6 A. W. Crosby, *The Columbian Exchange: The Biological and Cultural Consequences of 1492*, Westport, Conn., 1974; W. H. McNeill, *Plagues and Peoples*, Harmondsworth, 1979.

7 For some Indian examples see, I. D. Mills, 'The 1918–19 influenza pandemic: the Indian experience', *Indian Economic and Social History Review*, 23, 1986, pp. 1-40; T. Dyson (ed.), *India's Historical Demography: Studies in Famine, Disease and Society*, London, forthcoming. A useful collection of papers on medical anthropology is D. Landy (ed.), *Culture, Disease, and Healing: Studies in Medical Anthropology*, New York, 1977.

8 C. E. Rosenberg, 'George Rosen and the social history of medicine', in C. E. Rosenberg (ed.), *Healing and History*, Folkestone, 1979, p. 3. Cf., F. F. Cartwright, *A Social History of Medicine*, London, 1977, p. 1: 'The primary purpose of a social history of medicine must be to describe how the practice of medicine has affected the health and development of people.'

9 Quoted in E. Cook, *The Life of Florence Nightingale*, II, London, 1914, p. 1.

10 J. J. McKelvey, *Man against Tsetse: Struggle for Africa*, Ithaca, 1973, pp. 19-21. See, too, the discussion of western medical missions as a 'reconstructive force' in late nineteenth-century China in R. H. Graves, *Forty Years in China*, Baltimore, 1895, chapter 14.

11 Quoted in C. D. Langen's introduction to D. Schoute, *Occidental Therapeutics in the Netherlands East Indies during Three Centuries of Netherlands Settlement (1600–1900)*, Batavia, 1937, p. iii.

12 Quoted in J. Paul 'Medicine and imperialism in Morocco', *MERIP Reports*, 60, 1977, p. 7.

13 Quoted in Patterson, 'Disease and medicine', p. 148.

14 E.g., J. Suret-Canale, *French Colonialism in Tropical Africa, 1900–1945*, London, 1971, pp. 395-416.

15 D. Joralemon, 'New World depopulation and the case of disease', *Journal of Anthropological Research*, 38, 1982, pp. 108-27; Crosby, *Columbian Exchange*, chapter 2.

16 R. Elphick and H. Giliomee (eds.), *The Shaping of South African Society, 1652–1820*, London, 1979, pp. 22-3; A. W. Crosby, *Ecological Imperialism: The Biological Expansion of Europe, 900-1900*, Cambridge, 1986, chapters 9 and 10; D. Morley, 'Severe measles', and M. Kamien, 'The Aboriginal Australian experience', in N. F. Stanley and R. A. Joske (eds.), *Changing Disease Patterns and Human Behaviour*, London, 1980, pp. 117, 256.

17 Quoted in A. Moorehead, *The Fatal Impact: An Account of the Invasion of the South Pacific, 1767–1840*, Harmondsworth, 1966, p. 212.

18 R. Lange, 'Plagues and pestilences in Polynesia: the nineteenth-century Cook Islands experience', *Bulletin of the History of Medicine*, 58, 1984, p. 332.

19 'The sacrifice of human lives resulting from the global spread of pathogenic agents during these three centuries [1300–1600] has had no parallel before or since': E. Le Roy Ladurie, *The Mind and Method of the Historian*, Brighton, 1981, p. 30.

20 E.g., in Equatorial Africa and the Congo: Suret-Canale, *French Colonialism*, pp. 36-7; O. Ransford, *'Bid the Sickness Cease': Disease in the History of Black Africa*, London, 1983, p. 76. Disease was not the only cause of the massive population decreases recorded, but equally military conquest, coercive labour policies, and the disruption of agricultural production also contributed to the depopulation of early Spanish America.

21 Patterson and Hartwig, 'The disease factor', p. 4. India, too, may have reached a peak of mortality at about this time: see I. Klein, 'Death in India, 1871–1921', *Journal of Asian Studies*, 32, 1973, pp. 639-59.

22 Lange, 'Plagues and pestilence', pp. 326-9.

23 E.g., the jigger-flea from South America to Africa: see H. Kjekshus, *Ecology Control and Economic Development in East African History: The Case of Tanganyika, 1850–1950*, London, 1977, pp. 134-6.

24 I. R. Phimister, 'The "Spanish" influenza pandemic of 1918 and its impact on the Southern Rhodesian mining industry', *Central African Journal of Medicine*, 19, 1973, pp. 143-6; J. W. Brown, 'Increased intercommunication and epidemic disease in early colonial Ashanti', in Hartwig and Patterson, *Disease in African History*, p. 191.

25 J. M. de Figueiredo, 'Ayurvedic medicine in Goa according to European sources in the sixteenth and seventeenth centuries', *Bulletin of the History of Medicine*, 58, 1984, p. 227; M. J. Azevedo, 'Epidemic disease among the Sara of Southern Chad, 1890–1940', in Hartwig and Patterson, *Disease in African History*, p. 134.

26 Notably in East Africa during the First World War: A. Beck, *A History of the British Medical Administration of East Africa, 1900–1950*, Cambridge, Mass., 1970, p. 59-64.

27 M. W. De Lancey, 'Health and disease on the plantations of Cameroon, 1884–1939', in Hartwig and Patterson, *Disease in African History*, pp. 153-79; I. R. Phimister, 'African labour conditions and health in the Southern Rhodesian mining industry, 1898–1953', in I. R. Phimister and C. van Onselen, *Studies in the History of African Mine Labour in Colonial Zimbabwe*, Gwelo, 1987; R. M. Packard, 'Tuberculosis and the development of industrial health policies on the Witwatersrand, 1902–1932', *Journal of Southern African Studies*, 13, 1987, p. 186.

28 I. Klein, 'Malaria and mortality in Bengal, 1840–1921', *Indian Economic and Social History Review*, 9, 1972, pp. 132-60.

29 J. Ford, *The Role of Trypanosomiases in African Ecology: A Study of the Tsetse Fly Problem*, Oxford, 1971, p. 489. See also Kjekshus, *Ecology Control*.

30 T. O. Pearce, 'Political and economic changes in Nigeria and the organisation of medical care', *Social Science and Medicine*, 14, 1980, p. 95.

31 B. D. Paul, 'The role of beliefs and customs in sanitation programmes', in Landy, *Culture, Disease, and Healing*, p. 235.

32 N. Wachtel, *The Vision of the Vanquished: The Spanish Conquest through Indian Eyes, 1530–1570*, New York, 1977; D. Arnold, 'Cholera and colonialism in British India', *Past and Present*, 113, 1986, pp. 128-31.

33 Le Roy Ladurie, *Mind and Method of the Historian*, p. 29.

34 J. Orley, 'Indigenous concepts of disease and their interaction with scientific medicine', in E. E. Sabben-Clare, D. J. Bradley and K. Kirkwood (eds.), *Health in Tropical Africa during the Colonial Period*, Oxford, 1980, pp. 127-37.

35 Arnold, 'Cholera', pp. 140-2. Mental illness also occasioned extreme views of the 'native' mind and character: M. Vaughan, 'Idioms of madness: Zomba lunatic asylum, Nyasaland, in the colonial period', *Journal of Southern African Studies*, 9, 1983, pp. 218-38.

36 R. E. Dumett, 'The campaign against malaria and the expansion of scientific, medicial, and sanitary services in British West Africa, 1898–1910', *African Historical*

Studies, 1, 1968, p. 71; L. Spitzer, 'The mosquito and segregation in Sierra Leone', *Canadian Journal of African Studies*, 2, 1968, pp. 49-61; M. W. Swanson, 'The sanitation syndrome: bubonic plague and urban native policy in the Cape colony, 1900–1909', *Journal of African History*, 18, 1977, pp. 387-410.

37 McKelvey, *Man against Tsetse*, pp. 7-8; cf., Ronald Ross, *Memoirs*, London, 1923, p. 43, for malaria as a cause of Indians' 'great timidity', 'habit of unquestioning obedience' and 'amazingly deliciate physique'.

38 Crosby, *Ecological Imperialism*.

39 P. D. Curtin, '"The White Man's Grave": image and reality, 1780-1850', *Journal of British Studies*, 1, 1961, pp. 94-110; T. Wilkinson, *Two Monsoons*, London, 1976; H. Furber, *Rival Empires of Trade in the Orient, 1600–1800*, Minneapolis, 1976, p. 6.

40 F. Guerra, 'The influence of disease on race, logistics and colonisation in the Antilles', *Journal of Tropical Medicine and Hygiene*, 69, 1966, p. 34.

41 W. B. Cohen, 'Malaria and French imperialism', *Journal of African History*, 24, 1983, pp. 23-36.

42 G. Burke and P. Richardson, 'The profits of death: a comparative study of miners' phthisis in Cornwall and the Transvaal, 1876–1918', *Journal of Southern African Studies*, 4, 1978, p. 169. In Fiji indentured Indian labourers were brought in to work the sugar estates when the native Fijians were hit by the 1875 measles epidemic: Morley, 'Severe measles', p. 117.

43 D. R. Headrick, *Tools of Empire: Technology and European Imperialism in the Nineteenth Century*, New York, 1981, chapter 3.

44 Ransford, *'Bid the Sickness Cease'*, p. 71, though significantly the reference here is to the period from the 1880s.

45 Dumett, 'Campaign against malaria', pp. 155-7.

46 Cohen, 'Malaria', pp. 25-8; M. Gelfand, *Lakeside Pioneers: Socio-medical Study of Nyasaland (1850–1920)*, Oxford, 1964, pp. 11-14.

47 L. J. and J. M. Bruce-Chwatt, 'Malaria and yellow fever', in Sabben-Clare, *Health in Tropical Africa*, p. 58.

48 D. G. Crawford, *A History of the Indian Medical Service, 1600–1913*, I, London, 1914, pp. 113-28; for early Dutch medicine and hospitals at Batavia and the Cape, see Schoute, *Occidental Therapeutics*, and E. H. Burrows. *A History of Medicine in South Africa up to the End of the Nineteenth Century*, Cape Town, 1958, chapters 1 to 5.

49 C. S. Kidwell, 'Aztec and European medicine in the New World, 1521–1600', in L. Romanucci-Ross, D. E. Moerman, and L. R. Tancredi (eds,), *The Anthropology of Medicine: From Culture to Method*, New York, 1983, pp. 20-31; de Figueiredo, 'Ayurvedic medicine'. The Portuguese physician Garcia d'Orta at Goa in the sixteenth century and the Dutch Jacobus Bontius in Java in the seventeenth both studied and wrote major works about local drugs and medical practices.

50 Crawford, *Indian Medical Service*, I, p. 22.

51 E.g., among the Boers: Burrows, *Medicine in South Africa*, pp. 190-4.

52 J. Z. Bowers, 'The odyssey of smallpox vaccination', *Bulletin of the History of Medicine*, 55, 1981, pp. 17-33.

53 O. Temkin, *The Double Face of Janus*, Baltimore, 1977, p. 48.

54 Dumett, 'Campaign against malaria', p. 163; Michael Worboys, 'The emergence of tropical medicine: a study in the establishment of a scientific speciality', in G. Lemaine, R. MacLeod, M. Mulkay and P. Weingart (eds.), *Perspectives on the Emergence of Scientific Disciplines*, Hague, 1976, pp. 75-98. For the professionalisation of medicine in the United States during this period and its relationship with industrial capitalism, see E. R. Brown, *Rockefeller Medicine Men: Medicine and Capitalism in America*, Berkeley, 1979, pp. 74 f.

55 Swanson, 'Sanitation syndrome', and my chapter below; for developments in state medicine in Britain in this period, see J. L. Brand, *Doctors and the State: The British Medical Profession and Government Action in Public Health, 1870–1912*, Baltimore, 1965.

56 See Burrows, *Medicine in South Africa*, for the involvement of Dr W. G. Atherstone in various aspects of South African public life; and T. Ranger, 'The mobilisation of labour and the production of knowledge: the antiquarian tradition in Rhodesia', *Journal of African History*, 20, 1979, pp. 507-24, for the doctor, oral historian and ethnologist J. Blake-Thompson; and, more generally, Paul, 'Medicine and imperialism'.

57 McKelvey, *Man against Tsetse*, pp. 71-84; A. J. Duggan, 'Sleeping sickness epidemics', in Sabben-Clare, *Health in Tropical Africa*, pp. 19-29.

58 G. M. Gibson, *Physician to the World: The Life of General William Crawford Gorgas*, New York, 1950; A. J. Ornstein and J. Le Prince, *Mosquito Control in Panama*, New York, 1916. See also Reynaldo Ileto's chapter in this volume.

59 Schoute, *Occidental Therapeutics*, pp. 41, 165-7; Burrows, *Medicine in South Africa*, pp. 64-6.

60 W. Nitisastro, *Population Trends in Indonesia*, Ithaca, 1970, p. 41; Burrows, *Medicine in South Africa*, pp. 102-3, 121-2. As late as 1892, one West African Governor professed himself 'in perfect ignorance of sickness and mortality among tribes of the interior': Dumett, 'Campaign against malaria', p. 154.

61 Quoted in J. W. Cell, 'Anglo-Indian medical theory and the origins of segregation in West Africa', *American Historical Review*, 91, 1986, p. 321. As both Waltraud Ernst and John Farley show, 'poor whites' were also a major source of colonial concern if only for reasons of racial prestige.

62 W. Coleman, 'Epidemiological method in the 1860s: yellow fever at Saint-Nazaire', *Bulletin of the History of Medicine*, 58, 1984, pp. 161-3. As the work of Koch and Haffkine on cholera and its prophylaxis indicate, Europe used overseas territories like Egypt and India as laboratories for the investigation of diseases that still threatened Europe itself. The French (notably under Laveran) similarly used Algeria for research into a malaria that still menaced Mediterranean Europe, and yellow fever was a cause of concern in the United States long before the Havana and Panama campaigns at the turn of the century. In 1892, the year Haffkine presented his initial work on cholera prophylaxis in Paris, the disease was raging in the city. It was only because he was barred from conducting further tests in his native Russia that Haffkine turned to India instead in 1893–6 and so became involved in 'tropical' medicine: G. H. Bornside, 'Waldemar Haffkine's cholera vaccines and the Ferran-Haffkine priority dispute', *Journal of the History of Medicine*, 37, 1982, pp. 404-5.

63 N. Howard-Jones, *The Scientific Background of the International Sanitary Conferences, 1851–1938*, Geneva, 1975, pp. 74, 78-9.

64 McKelvey, *Man against Tsetse*, pp. 40-2; H. G. Soff, 'Sleeping sickness in the Lake Victoria region of British East Africa, 1900–1915', *African Historical Studies*, 2, 1969, p. 261; and Maryinez Lyons' chapter below.

65 Doyal, *Political Economy*, chapter 7; M. Gelfand, *A Service to the Sick: A History of the Health Services for Africans in Southern Rhodesia (1890–1953)*, Gwelo, 1976, pp. 17-18, 28, 36, 40; Beck, *British Medical Administration*, p. 73.

66 'The ravages of the tsetse-fly are the greatest menace to the development of tropical Africa', reported the East African Commission of 1925: Ford, *Role of Trypanosomiases*, p. 1; Worboys, 'Tropical medicine', p. 83-5; Dumett, 'Campaign against malaria', pp. 167-84. See, too, Michael Worboys' discussion of nutrition below.

67 Brown, *Rockefeller Medicine Men*, pp. 105-29. 'The Rockefeller programmes did not concern themselves with worker's physical productivity alone. They were also intended to reduce the cultural resistance of "backward" and "uncivilised" peoples to the domination of their lives and societies by industrial capitalism.' E. R. Brown, 'Public health in imperialism: early Rockefeller programs at home and abroad', *American Journal of Public Health*, 66, 1976, p. 900.

68 Schoute, *Occidental Therapeutics*, p. 189.

69 See my essay on smallpox vaccination below; Burrows, *Medicine in South Africa*, pp. 180-2 for the 'conquest by civilisation' policy in New Zealand and South Africa.

70 Quoted in Gelfand, *Lakeside Pioneers*, p. 8. The evangelical value of medical work had been appreciated in India and China at a slightly earlier date than in tropical

Africa – between the 1830s and 1850s. See I. H. Hacker, *A Hundred Years in Travancore, 1806–1906*, London, 1908, chapter 6; E. V. Gulick, *Peter Parker and the Opening of China*, Cambridge, Mass., 1973.

71 Gelfand, *Lakeside Pioneers*, p. 307; Burrows, *Medicine in South Africa*, p. 181. T. O. Ranger, 'Godly medicine: the ambiguities of medical mission in southeast Tanzania', *Social Science and Medicine*, 15, 1981, p. 262.

72 Ranger, 'Godly medicine'; P. C. G. Adams, 'Disease concepts among Africans in the Protectorate of Northern Rhodesia', *Rhodes-Livingstone Journal*, 10, 1950, pp. 14-50.

73 See also Duggan, 'Sleeping sickness', pp. 21-3; D. Arnold, 'Touching the body: perspectives on the Indian plague, 1896–1900', in R. Guha (ed.), *Subaltern Studies*, V, Delhi, 1987, pp. 55-90.

74 Quoted by R. W. Lieban, 'The field of medical anthropology', in Landy, *Culture, Disease, and Healing*, p. 14.

75 G. Maclean, 'Medical administration in the tropics', *British Medical Journal*, 1, 1950, p. 759.

76 Brown, *Rockefeller Medicine Men*, p. 75; Temkin, *Double Face of Janus*, pp. 435-6; Turshen, *Political Ecology*, pp. 11-16.

77 Paul, 'Medicine and imperialism', p. 8; G. W. Hartwig, 'Smallpox in the Sudan', *International Journal of African Historical Studies*, 14, 1981, pp. 15-16.

78 S. Ofusu-Amaah, 'The African experience', in Stanley and Joske, *Changing Disease Patterns*, p. 312; J. H. Ricosse, 'French West and Equatorial Africa', in Sabben-Clare, *Health in Tropical Africa*, pp. 228-38; McKelvey, *Man against Tsetse*, pp. 126 f.

79 F. Fanon, *A Dying Colonialism*, Harmondsworth, 1970, pp. 104-9.

80 Quoted in Beck, *British Medical Administration*, p. 84; cf., my chapter below.

81 I. J. Catanach, 'Plague and the Indian village, 1896–1914', in P. Robb (ed.), *Rural India: Land, Power and Society under British Rule*, London, 1983, pp. 216-43, and his essay in this volume; Arnold, 'Touching the body'. Two other inhibiting factors were important. One was the many technical difficulties that confronted western medicine in the tropics, even in such relatively simple matters as vaccination: Brown, 'Increased intercommunication', p. 189, and my chapter. Another critical factor was the unwillingness of most imperial governments to fund large-scale preventive campaigns. To his lasting chagrin, Ross was never allowed to conduct an imperial campaign against malaria-carrying mosquitoes with the kind of resources used by the Americans in Cuba and Panama: Dumett, 'Campaign against malaria', pp. 166-7, 189-90.

82 Beck, *British Medical Administration*, pp. 24-35; Worboys, 'Tropical medicine', pp. 90-1.

83 Beck, *British Medical Administration*, pp. 105 f.

84 A. Richards, *Land, Labour and Diet in Northern Rhodesia: An Economic Study of the Bemba Tribe*, Oxford, 1939, especially the introduction and chapter 3, 'Native views on food'. See, too, the special issue on 'African native diet', in *Africa*, 11, 1936.

85 E.g., Roger Jeffrey, 'Doctors and Congress: the role of medical men and medical politics in Indian nationalism', in M. Shepperdson and C. Simmons (eds.), *The Indian National Congress and the Political Economy of India 1885–1985*, Aldershot, 1988, pp. 160-73.

CHAPTER TWO

The European insane in British India, 1800–1858: a case-study in psychiatry and colonial rule

Waltraud Ernst

The rise of the European lunatic asylum

European efforts to establish psychiatric institutions in India date back to the eighteenth century. Provision for the confinement of the mentally ill was first made in Calcutta some time prior to 1787.[1] In 1794 the 'Madras Lunatic Asylum' was opened in order to afford 'security against the perpetration of those acts of violence which had been so frequently committed by unrestrained lunatics'.[2] By the late 1850s the number of establishments for the mentally ill, called 'Lunatic Asylums' or 'Hospitals for the Insane', had greatly multiplied. Each of the presidency towns of Calcutta, Bombay and Madras could boast its own 'asylum for the European insane'; about twenty 'native lunatic asylums' had been established in provincial towns, while the mentally ill in small stations were confined to various local jails or hospitals.[3] In contrast to the earlier decades, by the 1850s, European patients in the presidency towns were no longer sent to private establishments specialising in what had become notorious in England as the 'private trade in lunacy'. Rather, asylums for the European insane had gradually become specialist public institutions, supervised by European medical officers, and owned, financially maintained and controlled by the government authorities in Calcutta, Madras, and Bombay.

Along with the progressive expansion of European psychiatric institutions in India went a steady increase in the number of patients treated as mentally ill. The average number of patients confined in the European wards in the three main institutions in Calcutta, Madras and Bombay had been about fifty in 1820: by the 1850s it was almost double that number.[4] But although the number of asylums for Indians and Europeans and the number of asylum inmates appears to have increased over the decades, it must be stressed that this trend did not represent a 'great confinement', comparable to that alleged by Foucault to have occurred in Europe at this time.[5] Firstly, twenty or so asylums for the whole of India's vast area and population is a small figure when set against the estimated ninety psychiatric institutions in the British Isles in the 1850s. Secondly, the number of asylum inmates in British India was miniscule compared to the overall size of the population at the time and contrasts markedly with the very high percentage of people institutionalised in Britain in the late nineteenth and early twentieth centuries.[6] Even asylum architecture in British India bore silent testimony to the relative insignificance of psychiatric confinement there. Unlike the presidency towns' new general hospitals, built in the then highly acclaimed classical temple style, the asylums owed more to the less representative army-barrack design. Neither statistically nor in terms of the asylum's visual and symbolic representation could any Benthamite vision of the European lunatic panopticon be evoked.

In terms of the inmates' daily routine, too, the European lunatic asylum was no 'total institution' either. While the treatment of patients varied considerably according to the superintendent's ideas and disposition and the patients' social class, European inmates generally enjoyed some freedom to move about their wards, to find amusement in reading books and newspapers or playing cards, in wandering along the beach at Bombay or strolling in the garden in Calcutta. Admittedly, patients in Bombay and Calcutta enjoyed more salubrious surroundings than those in Madras, being housed in less dilapidated buildings. But even in Madras those Europeans who were by the 1840s still admitted to the then derelict asylum could enjoy considerable diversion, and the spatial constraints made possible greater freedom of contact between inmates of different cultural backgrounds.

Another factor which contributed to the relatively low-key character of psychiatric confinement in colonial India was the fact that psychiatry had not yet been separated from general medicine. The medical officer in charge of the presidency asylum had various additional responsibilities, such as being the civil surgeon, the superintendent of local dispensaries and jail hospitals, and he often had an extensive private practice. Apart from the consequent diffusion of his time and interest, his office as asylum superintendent was seen as less urgent and important than the treatment of fevers, cholera, and other widespread diseases. The persistent threat of disease contributed to the increasingly high status afforded to medical officers in India. It was, however, for those more common ailments rather than the less frequent cases of mental illness that the practitioner's services were most highly valued. The report of the Royal Commission on the Sanitary

State of the Army in India revealed in 1863 that the main causes of death among British soldiers in India between 1830 and 1846 were dysentery and diarrhoea (thirty-two per cent), 'fevers' (twenty-three per cent), diseases of the liver (ten per cent), and cholera (ten per cent).[7] These, in consequence, constituted the army's main enemy: only six per cent of European soldiers were killed in action or died of their wounds, while eighty-two per cent succumbed to disease within a twenty-year period of service in India. By comparison the incidence of 'insanity' as a cause of death was negligible. It amounted to a fraction of one per cent.[8]

In view of the relative insignificance of psychiatric confinement in British India (in terms of the small numbers involved and the existence of more pressing medical priorities), its role in maintaining the colonial 'order of things' might be questioned. The effect of psychiatric institutionalisation may have been highly significant for the individual concerned, but it would seem to have been devoid of any wider social impact among the majority of the colonisers and the colonised. The effectiveness of such confinement as an instrument for enforcing social discipline would indeed appear negligible if psychiatry were considered in isolation. However, if it is set within the broader context of colonial administration a different picture emerges.

The colonial order

By the beginning of the nineteenth century the British presence in India was no longer based exclusively on a trading interest. The battle of Plassey in 1757 and the granting of the *diwan* (governorship) of Bengal, Bihar and Orissa in 1765 to the English East India Company, as well as Pitt's India Act of 1784 and the momentous administrative reforms carried out during Cornwallis's term of office as Governor-General (1786–93), were decisive preconditions for the progressive transformation and consolidation of the Company's presence in India as a ruling power. The Company was made accountable to Parliament on the one hand while on the other it gradually assumed such state functions as revenue collection, judicial administration and responsibility for public welfare. Indians were no longer trading partners: they had become colonial subjects obliged to acknowledge British rule, even if the Company made some cultural and administrative concessions through a policy of 'indirect rule'. Along with the Company's evolution from trading enterprise to state organisation went the need to enforce and legitimate its newly assumed power.

A number of critical accounts exist which analyse the character and working of colonial rule as it was imposed on the people of India. Accounts of how notions of 'law and order' were enforced among Europeans themselves are, by contrast, scarce and more often anecdotal or literary than analytical in nature. And yet both the maintenance of discipline among European troops and the preservation of public peace among European civilians were a major preoccupation of colonial rule.

The Europeans in India were not a homogeneous community but were rather divided along lines of social class and national or regional origin, presided over by what has aptly been labelled a 'middle class aristocracy'.[9] This European elite, though mainly middle-class in origin, assumed in India an air of aristocratic exclusiveness, maintaining an ostentatious life-style and upper-class manners. The majority of Europeans, however, belonged to the lower classes. Their manners were often regarded as obnoxious by the European elite. It was argued that not only would their 'low and licentious' behaviour tend to 'vex, harass and perplex the weak natives',[10] but that it would also be detrimental to the maintenance of British rule in India. A 'spectacle' such as 'needy and reckless Europeans wandering about' the country was seen to be 'humiliating to the British character' and it was consequently urged that the government make arrangements by which 'fellow country men however degenerate, may cease by this public and humiliatory exhibition of these vices to dishonour here the country from which they spring'.[11]

The oft-asserted 'superiority of the European character' and the proclaimed enlightened spirit of British civilisation were considered vital to the legitimacy of colonial rule.[12] It is questionable whether the 'natives' would unreservedly have endorsed the British self-image of superiority and the concomitant belief that it was upon 'this feeling of the superiority of the Europeans' that the empire in India depended.[13] Whether reciprocated or not, the colonial ideology of European superiority undoubtedly contributed not only to the consolidation of British rule over Indians but also to the policing of Europeans within India. The grip of colonialism was thus tightened in respect of indigenous subjects and lower-class Europeans alike.

On the margins of European society

In the absence of a colonial equivalent of the English Poor Law, various alternative arrangements were made for the disciplining and social relief of those seen as deviant, delinquent and distressed Europeans. One part of this 'problem' of control was specific to the army and, to a degree, could be dealt with through military procedures. Minor breaches of army discipline were met with such punishment as extended drill and loss of leave while the 'most disgraceful and highly irregular conduct and neglect of duty to the prejudice of good order and discipline' was punishable by courts martial and subsequent incarceration, flogging or shooting. The line between a disciplinary measure's deterrent effect and the provocation of mutinous action or desertion seems always to have been a thin one. The high number of desertions from both the Company Army and from regiments of the British Army stationed in India provides evidence for this. Deserters may in part have been impelled by a longing for adventure in a foreign land, but the harsh nature of the army regulations themselves contributed to the decision to desert, especially when soldiers 'saw so many flogged' that they grew 'heartily tired of soldiering'.[14] Once former soldiers left military stations and began to roam about the country they attracted the attention of civil authorities and political agents. Although it was said that 'pecuniary aid is easily given in these cases', it was at the same time pointed out that the core of the problem created by European vagrancy and destitution was rather one of 'lowering the European character in the eyes of Natives'.[15] The government was repeatedly asked to provide against former soldiers, who, wandering 'throughout the country like wretched outcasts in search of food and liquor', 'ultimately fall victims to drunkenness, despair and a burning climate'.[16]

Among sailors, too, distress and vagrancy were widespread and often related to their terms of employment and current discharge practices. Like the soldiers, they were 'very little cared for by those whom they served'.[17] Sailors, however, tended to restrict their wanderings to the vicinity of sea ports. This did not please European residents, who early in the nineteenth century had begun to organise themselves through urban pressure groups and fund-raising bodies to improve the quality of life in what they regarded as *their* towns. Streets were widened, parks laid out, promenades watered and crowded 'native' market places moved elsewhere.[18] Against such a background of urban improvement, European vagrancy was seen both as harmful to the European rulers' prestige and as a blight on the city's elegance and beauty. The establishment of sailors' homes and hospitals funded by private subscriptions was partly inspired by such considerations. The Bombay Sailors' Home, for example, was established by private subscription following a shipwreck in 1836 which had left a number of sailors unprovided for and with no alternative but to beg in the streets until they could find work on another vessel. To the resident Europeans it seemed preferable to raise funds for relief in this manner than to suffer the alternative of destitute 'poor whites' roaming about the town.[19] A virtue could be made of this financial outlay by regarding it as a charitable contribution for the relief of 'suffering humanity'.[20]

What, then, was the importance of psychiatric institutions within the context of military discipline and the prevention of breaches of public order in civilian settlements?

The enforcement of army discipline and measures against European vagrancy on the one hand and the institutionalisation of European 'lunatics' on the other were closely interrelated. In many cases those classified as insane had a prior history of being court-martialled or of being confined in civil or military jails for crimes committed, or on vagrancy charges following their desertion or discharge from the army or navy. Considered a disruptive element in other institutions, their transference to a lunatic asylum was seen as a welcome solution by the civil and military authorities.

Gunner F. Harvey, for example, was sent to the Bombay Lunatic Asylum after having 'suddenly without any previous warning . . . sprung upon one of the men who was put upon watch' in the house of correction where he was confined.[21] Originally Harvey had been sentenced to a year's imprisonment for drunkenness and insubordination, but, due to his violent behaviour in the jail, he was removed to the asylum and eventually sent back to England. Harvey's transfer from the house of correction to the lunatic asylum was not a unique case. In newly annexed regions, such as the Punjab, where no psychiatric institutions had yet been built, the authorities soon came to feel that it was 'scarcely safe or prudent to keep criminal lunatics in our gaols where . . . no means exist for their safe custody or proper treatment'.[22] Even the confinement of the insane in jail hospitals was seen to be unsatisfactory. It was argued that it was 'objectionable', not as one might imagine, on account of the further distress and humiliation inflicted on the unfortunate mental patients by herding them in with criminals, but for two quite different reasons. Firstly, the noise made by the 'lunatics' disturbed the convicts: and secondly, and more significantly, the convicts, seeing that the insane were not held responsible for their acts, were tempted to feign insanity.[23] Putting the insane among convicts, it was concluded, was dangerous because the former 'set all discipline and subordination at defiance'.[24]

Even when the mentally ill were neither violent nor disruptive, confinement in an asylum was still seen to be advisable, notwithstanding the expense involved. European women, for example, who on their husband's or relative's death lost both livelihood and reason, were considered to be far better off within an asylum than out on the streets, where their behaviour and appearance were likely to offend the European community's sense of order and propriety. Joanah Kiernan had been in a 'distressed state of mind' from the time when her husband, a gunner in the Company's artillery, died. The couple had arrived in Madras in 1835 in the hope of making a better living than back home in Ireland where James Kiernan had been a labourer. Suddenly deprived of support by her husband's early death, Joanah and her three children faced a certain future of poverty in India unless relief was provided for them. When the children, two boys and a girl, were received into the Military Orphan Asylum in Madras, Joanah became 'so manifestly insane as to render it unsafe to leave her at large'. She was first taken to the General Hospital, but because of her continuing 'taciturn and dejected' state, she was later transferred to the Lunatic Asylum. Her 'insanity' was of a type shared by others of her gender: following the break-up of her family and the consequent loss of security and support, she became 'weak and depressed' and showed 'no interest in her children to whom she previously appeared to be much attached'. By remaining 'in the same state, generally appearing to understand what is said to her, but never uttering more than a single word in reply', Joanah Kiernan at least found relief for her children and an asylum regime of 'tonics and full diet' for herself.[25]

Two possible options available to the authorities in a case such as Mrs Kiernan's were either to discharge her from the asylum once her 'insane' behaviour had ceased or keep her inside the institution indefinitely. Both alternatives, however, ran counter to the government's policy of trying to curb European vagrancy and the Company Court of Director's order to restrict the hospitalisation of Europeans in India to a period of no more than a year. Mrs Kiernan was accordingly sent back to Britain. She died of bronchitis about fifty years later, at the age of seventy-eight, still confined to the Royal India Asylum, Ealing, where such 'insanes' from India were sent.[26]

The repatriation of asylum inmates thus conveniently removed the problem of European vagrancy from India and limited the expense of maintaining pauper patients in costly psychiatric institutions in India. Confinement in such institutions and subsequent transfer back to Britain can thus be seen as devices used by the colonial authorities in cases where a European's continued presence in India was seen to be highly disruptive or otherwise undesirable. Psychiatric confinement, which at first sight appears to be of only minor importance, thus assumes considerable importance within the wider context of the maintenance of colonial order and authority.

Inside the asylum

Despite its relative insignificance in quantitative terms, psychiatric provision for Europeans in India was an integral part of European social relief measures. The colonial society's values were in turn reflected in the way in which 'lunacy' policy was implemented. European civilisation, its spiritual aims and economic rationale, its institutions, technology, science and ideas, were seen to be paradigms for all human progress and moral development to follow. Consequently, 'those valuable improvements in the treatment of lunatics which have been introduced into European asylums' were transferred to British India in the firm conviction that there could not possibly exist any superior or more suitable arrangement.[27] In line with the social aspirations of a 'middle-class aristocracy' and the conviction that the British had a 'great moral duty to perform in India', strict class segregation was enforced within psychiatric institutions, along with discriminatory treatment for patients of different racial backgrounds.

As in England, the acknowledgement of and insistence upon distinct class divisions was a central feature of contemporary colonial society in India. The spirit of class-consciousness determined to a great extent the kinds of institutional settings and the quality of provision made available to members of the higher classes as to those from the lower ranks of white society. The rates charged for patients of various social strata, in India as much as in England, were elaborately graded in accordance with inmates' station in life. In the Calcutta Asylum, for example, prior to 1817, civil servants and 'gentlewomen' were maintained at the high rate of Rs 120 a month while pauper civilians had to make do with an eighth of that amount, a mere Rs 15. In a direct replication of the army and navy hierarchy, military employees were provided for according to their former rates of pay, which could have been as low as Rs 8 a month for an ordinary soldier. An exception was made in the case of 'independent gentlemen', who, though unconnected with the Company's service, were still considered eligible for a monthly rate of Rs 100 in recognition of their former social position.[28] These rates varied from presidency to presidency and over time. They were also not entirely undisputed as the Company's Court of Directors repeatedly pressed for a lowering of the expense of asylum inmates. Various reductions were made, but the principle of rates graded according to social class was, nevertheless, always strictly adhered to.

Patients' accommodation, being dependent on the maintenance rates, also varied considerably. In the Calcutta Lunatic Asylum the quarters of first-class patients were more spacious and comfortable than those available for lower-class inmates. The former lived in separate 'apartments': the latter were kept in the general 'wards'.[29] In the Madras Lunatic Asylum class-specific confinement among Europeans was also enforced during the earlier decades of the nineteenth century. There, however, the premises had become so derelict by the middle of the century and the lack of space so dire that the authorities refrained from sending higher-class patients to the asylum whenever alternative arrangements could be made for them. In 1851, for example, a Captain J. Campbell, who had been certified as a 'criminal lunatic', was not admitted to the asylum because it was regarded as 'unsuited for persons of his class'. Instead he was confined in the local prison, where he occupied a large part of the premises.[30] The prison staff continually complained about his presence there as not only did he take up much needed space, but he also 'most materially' upset prison discipline.[31]

Within the confined space of the Bombay Lunatic Asylum, by contrast, racial prejudice and social distance could be measured almost by the foot. The elaborate system of room allocation was based mainly on considerations of race, social status and gender, and only secondarily on medical grounds. The front wing of the building, which comprised the main entrance, the superintendent's quarters and some comfortably furnished rooms, was reserved for higher-class Europeans. The two-storeyed side wings accommodated patients of various descriptions, namely 'females of all castes and colour', 'European males', and 'native males'. The western wing, which overlooked the sea and contained the best rooms in the side wings, was allocated to the few lower-class Europeans that were confined in Bombay at any one time. The eastern wing was reserved exclusively for Indians and had to house as many as forty patients on each floor, whereas not more than about four inmates, on average, were accommodated in the second-class European ward. Thus both class discrimination and racial segregation were implemented within the confines of a single institution. While the Europeans' sea-facing wing commanded 'cheerful and pleasing views . . . of the entrance to the harbour, bay, Malabar Hill and the adjacent country', the 'native wings' were in such a miserable state that, according to the medical superintendent, it was 'not little short of a miracle that a man ever leaves this hospital cured'.[32]

Despite some variation in the enforcement of intra-institutional segregation, social class and racial background were the main determinants of room allocation within the three main asylums in British India. Similarly, the dietary regimes and provision of general services were also made in accordance with patients' class and race – so much so that cure and mortality rates at the beginning of the century correlated significantly with patients' social standing and in particular with their food provision. In the period from 1824 to 1850, for example, the mortality rate in the Calcutta Asylum amounted to 4.1 per cent in the case of first-class and 7.7 per cent in the case of second-class European patients.[33] This 'circumstance of the mortality of the second-class patients being nearly double that of the first-class patients' was considered 'very remarkable' by the authorities.[34] But, despite these findings, a few years later the asylum superintendent reduced the quantity of food provided for second-class patients, thereby achieving a decrease in monthly expenditure per patient of about Rs 4: the existing scale of provision for first-class patients was judged 'unexceptionable'.[35] Although experience in various asylums throughout the provinces had shown that food provision was a vital determinant of patients' mortality and cure rates, no effective recommendation was made by the presidency medical boards to ensure a full diet regime for lower-class inmates.

Patients' involvement in work and recreational activities, described as 'occupations which are incompatible with unhealthy mental excitement', was a main constituent of the contemporary system of 'moral treatment'.[37] The nature and availability of such activities again varied both with patients' social standing, race, and the constrictions of space in the different asylum premises. In the Bombay Asylum 'various household duties' as well as 'catalogue books, magazines and papers, backgammon, bagatelle, cards and chess, skittles and other out-of-door games' were mentioned as the 'principle instruments of moral treatment'.[38] As both Europeans and Indians were confined within the same compound, it was made clear that reading material such as *Punch* and the *Illustrated News* were meant for Europeans only. The exclusiveness of recreational facilities was, in this instance, based on racial, rather than class, considerations. Indians' amusements were to consist of 'ball, shooting with the bow, parhus, and one or two games of a like kind'.[39] Indian inmates were also allowed to keep pets at the institution, including dogs, cats, goats, fowls, pigeons, monkeys and deer. This peculiar practice had, according to the superintendent, been permitted 'with a view to calling out the gentler and kindlier feelings' of the patients.[40] Pastimes available to patients were thus in keeping with European preconceptions: the European inmates were encouraged to read, or to engage in the kinds of games that would be acceptable in polite English company; for Indians combative games and animal husbandry were regarded as more appropriate. The choice of pastimes thus reinforced the stereotype ideal of the European – superior in intellect and manners – as opposed to that of the typical Indian – given to fighting and accustomed to caring for animals. The activities may, of course, have been chosen with regard to the preferences of the European and Indian patients themselves, but a race-conscious ideology was also evident in the asylum administration's allocation of such pastimes.

Although the racial factor appears to have been decisive in the distribution of recreational activities in the Bombay Asylum, class divisions among European patients were no less important. But, due to the fact that the majority of European inmates belonged to the lower ranks of military employees while only a negligible number of patients each year were drawn from the higher classes, classification among the Europeans called for less elaboration. It went without saying that 'gentlemen' would be provided with all the amenities seen as fitting to their former station in life. The classificatory system therefore only needed further explication with regard to the lower-class Europeans' separation from Indians.

Institutional segregation, such as that practised in Bombay, may have facilitated efficient management and the comfort of the inmates; but at the same time the internal organisation of the institution was made in accordance with the same social priorities and prejudices prevailing in European society at large. Europeans of all ranks enjoyed a degree of comfort superior to that of Indians. Even in regard to the degree of consideration given to social background Europeans were preferentially treated. Their social sensitivities were respected and the lower ranks were duly separated from the higher. Indians' highly developed caste and religious sentiments, by contrast, were largely neglected. Indian males were huddled together and their institutional classification was made mainly on the basis of their symptomatic behaviour – whether they were quiet, of 'clean habits', violent or convalescent.[41] From a present-day point of view the seemingly egalitarian mode of classification applied to Indian inmates might appear preferable to the recreation within the asylum of outside patterns of social stratification. However, the neglect of Indians' differences of caste, class and creed derived from the Europeans' derogatory perception of all Indians as 'natives', as people of inferior race whose sensitivities and social prejudices could happily be ignored.

In the Calcutta Asylum, to which Indian patients were not usually admitted, social class was the main criterion for access to recreational facilities. During the 1820s, when the asylum was still managed by the proprietor of the building in which the patients were housed and when 'want of space and accommodation' was not yet felt,[42] first-class patients would occasionally have dinner with the superintendent's family or take their meals in the dining hall, which was comfortably provided with *punkahs* (ceiling fans). Access to the asylum library was similarly selective in the early period: later on this amenity was sacrificed to the need for further accommodation. In Calcutta, therefore, work and recreational facilities for the majority of patients became ever more constricted as a result of the growing overcrowdedness of the premises. By the middle of the century first-class patients were still provided with magazines and ward patients could spend most of the time during the day sitting on the verandahs, but voluntary labour, seen at the time as the 'most important remedial employment in asylums in Europe', was no longer available. Its absence in Calcutta was made a virtue of by the superintendent who claimed that it was 'utterly inapplicable in tropical India' and 'injurious to Europeans'. The climate was said to make 'farming, gardening and occupation in the kitchen, laundry or bakehouse impracticable'. It was also thought that 'mechanical labour would be uncongenial' to the 'majority of the patients', who were 'soldiers, sailors and gentlemen'.[43]

Clearly, then, despite some local variations, questions of social and racial origins were afforded great consideration in these institutions. Class divisions among Europeans were carefully preserved and reflected in the various provisions and amenities made available to the inmates. The staff employed in the asylums was hierarchically organised, too, and its stratification echoed the race, class and gender classification applied to the patients. The most senior position within the asylum was that of medical superintendent. As he was in medical and managerial charge of the institution he was invariably a European.[44] For European patients the services of European head keepers were provided.[45] No problem was apparently encountered in the recruitment of suitable persons for this work. Former soldiers and sailors, who preferred employment in India to a doubtful future back in Britain after many years abroad or who had married Indian women, could readily be found. There seems to have been greater difficulty, however, in finding suitable female head keepers. In order to qualify for the post of supervising the care of European women, the candidate had to be not only European, but also of a 'respectable' class and yet willing to accept the very low pay (about Rs 8 to 15 a month).[46] There also seems to have been a racial qualification for the post of assistant apothecary, but not for that of compounder.[47] The remaining employees, consisting of cooks, sweepers, watchmen, watercarriers, washermen, barbers and ward attendents, formed the asylum's 'native establishment'.[48] They were expected to 'shew the greatest deference and obedience to the subordinate officers' (usually Europeans) and to perform 'quietly' a wide range of menial and service tasks.[49]

While the number of European superior staff employed seems to have been lower than in private asylums in England, the European institutions in India were staffed with a considerably larger number of subordinate servants than was usual in private and public establishments in Europe. As the number of European personnel recommended in the 1820s remained stationary while the number of patients increased ten fold, it must have been the Indian servants who had to compensate for the declining standard of the general services.[50] Even so, the conditions in the European quarters in Bombay, where there was one attendant for every three Europeans, must have been superior to the 'native wards', where there was only one attendant for every seven Indians.[51]

Racial discrimination was openly advocated by the local authorities in India whenever the asylums' admission practices and general management came under scrutiny. When in 1820 the Calcutta Asylum's institutional arrangements were reviewed by the presidency's medical board and the Company's Court of Directors in London, the latter suggested that for reasons of economy the exclusively European asylum should be abolished and mentally ill Europeans should henceforth be sent to the newly established Native Lunatic Asylum.[52] The local authorities strongly objected to this proposal, arguing that 'the propriety of mixing Europeans labouring under mental derangement, with natives in the same condition [was] very questionable'.[53] Even the 'mixing' of lower-class Europeans with Indians was considered unacceptable. Consequently, a highly expensive separate establishment was maintained solely for the European insane.[54] In Madras and Bombay, however, there was a less stringent separation of the races. Europeans and Indians were confined within the same premises there, though still in segregated conditions.

Repatriation

The structure of a colonial society divided along lines of race and class could not but be reproduced within the institutional settings that society created. The existence of specialised establishments in turn provided for the assertion of organised state authority even over that society's marginal groups. The existence of a policy designed to complement the confinement of Europeans within psychiatric institutions in India – namely the transfer of mentally-ill Europeans back to Europe – serves to reinforce this point. The repatriation policy was established as a standard procedure in 1819, when the maximum term of confinement for Europeans in asylums in India was set at one year.[55] Calcutta, Madras and Bombay were the major ports for the embarkation of the European 'lunatics'. During the year they were sent in batches from the interior provinces and districts to the presidency towns, where they were received into the asylums for further observation. When recovery within a year seemed unlikely they were sent back to Europe.

This policy was adopted and retained for a number of practical as well as ideological reasons. To begin with, the maintenance of asylum establishments in India was very costly. House rents and land prices were chronically high, especially in Calcutta, as were salaries for European staff. More staff were needed in an asylum than in comparable institutions, such as prisons, where inmates could be conveniently locked away and guarded by Indian jailers. First-class asylums' inmates, it was felt, could not be deprived of their personal servants and attendants. Their mental state was not regarded as a terminal illness but rather as an affliction that might in time subside, enabling the patients to escape from their temporary misfortune and return to their former social environment. Even long-term first-class patients could not, it was believed, be justly deprived of their former privileges, although this might involve considerable expense. Lower-class Europeans were also thought to need the services of European attendants, but in their case the reason was the patients' commonly violent response to 'native' supervision as well as the authorities' determined opposition to the appointment of Indians to positions where they would have command over Europeans.[56] Considerations such as these tended to raise the cost of European establishments in India. A pragmatic way of saving money might have been the establishment of panopticon-style institutions of the kind then in vogue in Britain, where economies of scale could be applied.[57] But since such a solution would have necessitated the amalgamation of the relatively small European establishments with 'native' ones, it was never adopted. Instead the length of stay in these costly, small-scale institutions was restricted to a year and passages from India were provided for patients needing further care and treatment.

Another relevant aspect of the repatriation policy relates to the Company's concern to restrict white immigration into India. The assumed threat to the European rulers' prestige from the presence of distressed or other socially undesirable lower-class Europeans was an old argument, used against any possible colonisation of India by Europeans from the late eighteenth century onwards.[58] Following the Company's loss first of its Indian commercial monopoly in 1813 and then in 1833 of its exclusive trading rights with China, a restrictive immigration policy could no longer be as strictly adhered to. Nevertheless, various successful attempts were made to prevent discharged soldiers from staying on in India and to repatriate destitute Europeans. The sort of people the Company wanted in the East were civil and military officers who would set up profitable trading enterprises or in other ways further the cause of European rule, rather than people who would echo the lower-class misery and destitution of Britain itself or who, through sickness or personal tragedy, were unable to provide for themselves. Deportation of mentally ill Europeans thus fitted into the already established practice of controlling the European influx into India by shipping off home those seen as socially undesirable and economically unproductive.

Further, a patriotic and sentimental image of Britain's 'green and pleasant land' as the ultimate refuge and real home for British military and civil servants emerged alongside ideas of an overseas 'civilising' mission. The lower-classes' alleged lack of moral restraint and sense of duty was seen to be aggravated rather than diminished by service in the tropics. Once affected by the deleterious effects of exposure to the sun and to what was called 'hard living', Europeans' only chance of recovery was thought to rest in the early 'removal of those unfortunate persons to a colder climate',[59] as 'in no instance, after an attack of insanity should a man be permitted to remain in circumstances and relations which are obviously so likely to lead to a relapse'.[60]

The transfer of invalids, persons of 'bad character', the destitute and mentally ill can be traced back to well before 1800 when European immigration control emerged as part of a colonial policy of restricting the presence of lower-class Europeans in British India. Within this broader regulatory context the Company's policy towards 'lunatics' can be characterised as disposing of the problem by deporting the mentally ill themselves. At the same time the repatriation procedure contributed towards the strengthening of the contemporary ideological stance against cultural and racial integration, thereby countering any tendency for Europeans to 'go native'. Repatriation, as much as institutional segregation, served to maintain social distance between the various races and classes under the Company's rule in India.

Psychiatry and colonial rule

It would appear, then, that in the early nineteenth century psychiatry had become an integral part of the colonial system of social welfare and control. It also fulfilled an important ideological function, a role it held despite the limited use made of psychiatric confinement. The contemporary rhetoric of the lunatic asylum as a showpiece of British humanitarianism and scientific progress in India sounds overblown when set against the small number and scale of the institutions actually established. And yet it is exactly this overstatement, and the disproportionate claims made for psychiatry that helped to foster the self-image of the British as a race of humanitarian and rational rulers, whose scientific achievements endorsed claims for the benevolence and legitimacy of colonial rule. This legitimacy was to remain as fiercely contested as it was confidently asserted, and European psychiatry similarly remained an important symbolic marker for advocates and opponents of the continuing British presence in India. The ideological role of psychiatry outlived the end of the Company's administration in 1858 and persisted into the heyday of imperial rule when the confinement of European and Indian 'lunatics' in specialised institutions was implemented on a larger (though still restricted) scale. Of course, economic and political arguments can be advanced to explain colonial rule and its characteristic features. But the ideological pillars of colonialism were essential, too, to the preservation of its image and authority and are equally relevant to an understanding of its character. It is in this context that psychiatry can be seen to possess an importance that went far beyond its immediate role in controlling a few 'deviant' and 'harmful' individuals and in subjugating unreason.

Notes

1 D. G. Crawford, *A History of the Indian Medical Service*, II, London, 1914, p. 429.

2 Madras Military Letters, 18 February 1799, 88. All the archival sources cited in this article are located in the India Office Library and Records, London.

3 For a discussion of the East India Company's policy towards and provision for the Indian mentally ill, see W. Ernst, '"Native Lunatic Asylums" in early nineteenth-century British India', in G. J. Meulenbeld and D. Wujastek (eds.), *Studies in Indian Medical History*, Groningen, 1987.

4 The number of mentally ill persons deported to Britain and subsequently confined in asylums there was equally insignificant: for the statistics, see W. Ernst 'Psychiatry and Colonialism: The Treatment of the European Insane in British India, 1800–1858', unpublished Ph.D. thesis, University of London, 1986.

5 M. Foucault, *Madness and Civilization*, London, 1967 (first published 1961).

6 For psychiatric institutions in Europe, see K. Doerner, *Madmen and the Bourgeoisie: A Social History of Insanity and Psychiatry*, Oxford, 1969; R. Porter, 'The history of institutional psychiatry in Europe', in *The Yale Handbook of the History of Psychiatry*, forthcoming.

7 *Report of the Royal Commission on the Sanitary State of the Army in India*, London, 1863, p. XV.

8 *Sanitary State*, pp. XIII, 576: the estimate is taken from regimental statistics. The incidence rate of mental illness among Europeans in India was estimated to have been between one and two per cent: J. Macpherson, 'Lunatic asylums in Bengal'. *Calcutta Review*, XXVI, 1856, p. 603.

9 F. G. Hutchins, *The Illusion of Permanence: British Imperialism in India*, Princeton, 1967.

10 A. T. Embree, *Charles Grant and British Rule in India*, London, 1962, p. 169.

11 Political Letters from India, 5 September 1838, 69; Resident at Indore to Government of India, 31 October 1838, India Political Proceedings, 14 May 1838, 182. For a detailed analysis of European vagrancy, see D. Arnold, 'European orphans and vagrants in India in the nineteenth century', *Journal of Imperial and Commonwealth History*, VII, 1979, pp. 106–14.

12 Dundas, in *Hansard*, Parliamentary Debates (Commons), XXX, 23 April 1793, 676.

13 *Idem.* Cf. D. Arnold, 'White colonization and labour in nineteenth-century India', *Journal of Imperial and Commonwealth History,* XI, 1983, p. 139.
14 'A Grenadier's Diary, 1842–1856', 7 April 1846 [India Office manuscripts].
15 Resident, Indore, to Government of India, 31 October 1838, India Political Proceedings, 14 March 1838, 182.
16 *Ibid.*
17 'Grenadier's Diary', 25 June 1857.
18 See, for examples, J. B. Harrison, 'Allahabad: a sanitary history', and S. U. Ahmed, 'Urban problems and government policies: a case study of the city of Dacca, 1810–1830', in K. Ballhatchet and J. Harrison (eds.), *The City in South Asia: Pre-Modern and Modern,* London, 1980.
19 *City of Bombay Gazetteer,* III, Bombay, 1910.
20 J. Beardsmore to Government, 5 May 1836, Bengal Public Proceedings, 18 May 1836, 17.
21 Surgeon, House of Correction, report, 29 October 1852; Records of Pembroke House and Ealing Lunatic Asylum, medical certificates, 1853.
22 Minute, Medical Board, 29 August 1850, Bombay Public Proceedings, 9 October 1850, 7656.
23 C. J. Lodge Patch, *A Critical Review of the Punjab Mental Hospitals from 1840–1930,* Lahore, 1931, p. 9, quoting R. Montgomery, Judicial Commissioner.
24 Judicial Commissioner to Chief Commissioner, Punjab, 28 October 1853, in *Punjab Mental Hospitals,* para. 18.
25 Pembroke House and Ealing Lunatic Asylum, medical certificates, 1843.
26 *Ibid.*, case books, 1846–9, 1859–68, 1868–70, 1870–83, 1883–92. For a short description of the Royal India Asylum, Ealing, see W. Ernst and D. Kantowsky, 'Mad tales from the Raj: case studies from Pembroke House and Ealing Lunatic Asylum, 1818–1892', *Society,* XXII, 1985, pp. 31–8.
27 Bengal Public Despatches, 5 February 1851, 14.
28 Rates in the 'Government Lunatic Asylum' prior to 1817, referred to in Medical Board to Government, 20 October 1847, Bengal Public Proceedings, 21 June 1848, 6.
29 Asylum report, 14 June 1856, Bengal Public Proceedings, 24 June 1856, 52.
30 Chief Magistrate and Superintendent of Police to Military Board, 21 August 1852, Madras Judicial Letters, 30 October 1852, 2.
31 *Idem.*
32 Asylum Superintendent to Medical Board, 28 February 1850, Bombay Public Proceedings, 12 June 1852, 3815.
33 Medical Board to Government, 10 March 1851, Bengal Public Proceedings, 24 June 1852, 6.
34 Note by Secretary to Government, 9 June 1852, Bengal Public Proceedings, 24 June 1852, 9.
35 Asylum report, 14 June 1856, Bengal Public Proceedings, 24 June 1856, 52.
36 For the 'native lunatic asylums' in Bengal and the North-Western Provinces, see Ernst '"Native Lunatic Asylums"'. Note the contrast between the Bombay Asylum superintendent's comments on a diversified and liberal diet and the prevalence of scurvy (sixteen out of thirty-five patients suffered from this ailment) in the asylum: Asylum report, 31 March 1852, Medical Board to Government, 24 May 1853, Bombay Public Proceedings, 9 July 1853, 4537, Appendix, Table 2.
37 *Ibid.*, para. 73.
38 *Ibid.*, para. 74.
39 *Ibid.*, para. 76.
40 *Idem.*
41 Officially, Indians confined in European institutions should have been separated according to their ethnic, religious and caste background. Such segregation was, however, implemented only when 'practicable': in view of their overcrowded state such segregation in the Bombay and Madras asylums was scarcely 'practicable'. For further evidence, see Ernst, '"Native Lunatic Asylums"'; Ernst, 'Psychiatry and colonialism'.
42 Asylum report, 14 June 1856, Bengal Public Proceedings, 24 June 1856, 52.

43 *Idem.*
44 G. O. Medical Department: 'Half castes and other natives to be confined to subordinate offices': Bombay Military Despatches, 8 February 1826, 52.
45 Asylum report, 31 March 1852, Medical Board to Government, 24 May 1853, Bombay Public Proceedings, 9 July 1853, 4537.
46 Asylum report, 31 March 1850, Medical Board to Government, 23 August 1850, Bombay Public Proceedings, 9 October 1850, 7654A.
47 Asylum report, 31 March 1852, Medical Board to Government, 24 May 1853, Bombay Public Proceedings, 9 July 1853, 4537.
48 *Idem.*
49 Asylum report, 14 June 1856, Bengal Public Proceedings, 24 June 1856, 52.
50 Asylum report, Medical Board to Government, 23 August 1850, Bombay Public Proceedings, 9 October 1850, 7654A; Asylum report, 31 March 1852, Medical Board to Government, 24 May 1853, Bombay Public Proceedings, 9 July 1853, 4537.
51 Asylum report, 31 March 1850, Medical Board to Government, 23 August 1850, Bombay Public Proceedings, 9 October 1850, 7654A.
52 Bengal Public Despatches, 28 June 1820, 94.
53 Medical Board to Government, 5 February 1821, Bengal Public Proceedings, 20 February 1821, 32.
54 For an institutional history of the European Asylum at Bhowanipur, See Ernst, 'Psychiatry and colonialism'.
55 Public Letter from Bengal, 26 February 1819, 1.
56 The use of mechanical constraint was seen as preferable to physical coercion: 'Another consideration, which certainly ought not to be lost sight of, is the humiliation or the degradation to a European's feelings in being coerced by Natives'. Asylum report, 14 June 1856, Bengal Public Proceedings, 24 June 1856, 52; also, Bombay Military Despatches, 8 February 1826, 52.
57 In 1847 G. A. Berwick, M.D., suggested the establishment of a single 'Bengal Lunatic Asylum' which would be characterised by 'unity, simplicity of purpose, [and] economy', as both Indians and Europeans would be confined within a single compound: Berwick to Government, 5 March 1847, Bengal Public Proceedings, 26 May 1847, 123. This plan was described by the Medical Board of Bengal as a 'crude and incongruous scheme of assembling Europeans and Natives in one establishment': Medical Board to Government, 20 October 1847, Bengal Public Proceedings, 21 June 1848, 6.
58 Arnold, 'White colonization'.
59 Medical Board to Government, 30 November 1818, Bengal Public Proceedings, 4 December 1818, 18.
60 Pembroke House and Ealing Lunatic Asylum, medical certificates, 1852, case of H. Strauch.

CHAPTER THREE

Smallpox and colonial medicine in nineteenth-century India

David Arnold

To many nineteenth-century British medical officers smallpox was 'the scourge of India'. Reputedly 'one of the most violent and severe diseases to which the human race is liable', smallpox was held responsible for 'more victims than all other diseases combined', outstripping even cholera and plague in its 'tenacity and malignity'.[1] Several million deaths in the late nineteenth century alone were attributed to its destructive powers. Fatal in a third of all cases, smallpox also resulted in the permanent scarring and disfigurement of many of its survivors: one estimate blamed the disease for three-quarters of the blindness in India.[2]

But high mortality and lasting disability were not all that marked out smallpox as a disease of exceptional significance in nineteenth-century India. Smallpox occupied a distinctive place in both Indian and British attitudes to disease, curing and prevention. One of the most readily identifiable as well as one of the most virulent of India's epidemic diseases, smallpox was widely represented in religious belief and ritual, with smallpox deities worshipped throughout virtually the whole of India. The disease was also uniquely subject to human intervention. Jennerian vaccination, introduced to India in 1802, encouraged the British to regard smallpox as a preventible disease. At a time when the concerns of colonial physicians remained narrowly focused on European needs, vaccination represented a rare attempt to carry western medicine to the people. Indeed, it entailed a degree of state medical intervention unparalleled until the anti-plague campaigns of the late 1890s.[3] But, despite what the British saw as the indisputable benefits of vaccination, the practice was slow to gain general acceptance. One factor in this was the attitude of the colonial administration itself, especially with regard to carrying the costs entailed. There were practical difficulties to be overcome, too. But, in addition, vaccination was faced with the challenge of a rival prophylactic practice in inoculation and a rival agency in the indigenous variolators. Through a combination of these factors, it took a hundred years for vaccination to become an effective form of mass prophylaxis in India, and a further seventy years before the dread disease was finally eradicated.[4]

Partly because smallpox figured so prominently in British and Indian ideas about medicine and disease (and partly, too, because it was so extensively discussed in the medical literature of the time) smallpox offers valuable insights into the nature, purposes and impact of colonial medicine in India, and also, by reflection, into the interventionist capacities and practical limitations of colonial state power in India.

Disease and ritual in India

References to a pustular disease called *masurika* in Sanskrit medical texts dating back over two thousand years suggest that smallpox was an ancient affliction among the peoples of South Asia.[5] It is probable, however, that the virulence of the disease was not constant but fluctuated with differing viral strains and with changing human susceptibility. Ralph Nicholas has argued, mainly on the basis of literary sources, that smallpox was relatively mild in Bengal until, in the eighteenth century, Maratha raiding and British conquest disrupted rural society and caused the famines and population movements that favoured the dissemination of smallpox. He argues, too, that in these circumstances inoculation would have been neglected, thus removing a hitherto important check on its spread.[6] There is certainly evidence from more recent times of a close correlation between smallpox epidemicity on the one hand and famine and political dislocation on the other.[7]

Smallpox also followed a shorter and more predictable cycle. Endemic throughout most of India, the disease returned in epidemic strength every four to eight years with the creation of a pool of susceptible children born since the previous epidemic. In India the disease also showed a striking seasonality. It was so prevalent between February and May that it was widely known in eastern India as *basanta-roga*, the 'spring disease'.[8] With the onset of the monsoon season the disease declined, reaching its lowest annual ebb in October and November. Atmospheric conditions (the smallpox virus was more active and more readily transmissible in dry weather than in wet) offer a partial explanation for this pattern of occurrence. But social and cultural influences were important, too. In India the spring months were traditionally a time for congregation and travel. Pilgrimages to major shrines, popular religious fairs and marriage festivities were all most common during the dry part of the year when travel was easiest and little work was needed on the land. These activities provided the social mobility and contact necessary for smallpox transmission. Famines, in addition to weakening human resistance to infection, had a comparable effect: the famine-struck wandered in search of food or congregated in relief camps and towns where smallpox and other diseases were easily communicated.[9]

In the absence of detailed statistics before the 1880s, it is difficult to gauge the full extent of smallpox mortality in British India. It is possible that early estimates were greatly exaggerated. Because smallpox was a familiar disease and one greatly feared in Europe itself mortality may have been mistakenly attributed to it rather than to diseases that were then largely unknown. In Calcutta, for which some data exists, smallpox deaths averaged 734 a year between 1837 and 1865; but many fatal cases probably passed unrecorded in these early years. In the first five months of 1850, an epidemic year, there were 3,329 known deaths among the city's estimated 387,398 Indian inhabitants.[10] R. Pringle, writing in the *Lancet* in 1869, speculated that in the populous Doab tract of northern India as many as ninety-five per cent of the population may have been exposed to smallpox at some stage in their life. So prevalent was the disease, he added, that 'it has become quite a saying among the agricultural and even wealthier classes never to count children as permanent members of the family . . . until they have been attacked with and recovered from smallpox.'[11]

By the 1880s more reliable mortality statistics were being compiled in India, though recording procedures were still clearly deficient. By this date, too, vaccination may also have begun to have had some effect on reducing mortality from the disease. From 1.44 million deaths in the decade 1868–77 and 1.46 million in the decade 1878-1887, smallpox mortality fell to 0.96 million in 1888–97 and 0.83 million in 1898–1907.[12]

A major cause of Indian mortality, smallpox was also greatly feared among Europeans in India. Before 1800 British residents had some recourse to variolation (inoculation with smallpox matter), perhaps in emulation of current European rather than Indian practice. Otherwise they fled 'in terror' from their homes until the epidemic had passed.[13] With the rapid adoption of vaccination after 1802 Europeans became less vulnerable to smallpox than many other diseases encountered in India, such as cholera. But in the 1849–50 epidemic in Calcutta, seventy-six Europeans were taken to the city's General Hospital suffering from the disease and there were twenty fatalities. Most of the victims were 'poor Europeans', especially soldiers and sailors. Wealthier Europeans were thought to be protected not only by vaccination but also by the spaciousness of their houses and gardens and by the absence of close contact with Indians.[14]

Diminished susceptibility to the disease did not, however, mean that smallpox ceased to be a matter of European concern. Vaccination was sometimes so poorly performed as to be almost 'worthless' and until revaccination was introduced in the second half of the century immunity could be shortlived. Children were felt to be particularly at risk from Indian servants who might transmit the disease from their 'obscure homes in the bazaar'.[15] As late as 1893 one of the arguments used for compulsory vaccination in Pune (Poona) was 'in consideration of the proximity of the city to the large European population of the cantonment and the constant intercommunication which exists between the city and the cantonment'.[16] Since some degree of contact with the Indian population was unavoidable, one of the priorities of western medicine in India was to build a *cordon sanitaire* around the white community, with those Indians closest to it – domestic servants, soldiers, even plantation labourers – among the first to be singled out for vaccination. Demands that inoculation be prohibited and vaccination made compulsory were prompted first by a desire to protect European, rather than Indian, lives. Latterly, however, wider commercial and administrative considerations were involved, with European planters and factory owners seeing practical advantages in a vaccinated workforce.[17]

Most Europeans in nineteenth-century India held a secular view of smallpox and, in the later decades, took readily to the germ theory of disease causation. For the majority of Indians, however, smallpox bore a strong religious signification. Across a wide belt of India, from Bengal in the east to Maharashtra and Gujarat in the west, the goddess Sitala was identified as the deity responsible for bringing or preventing the disease. In southern India the goddess Mariyamma shared some of the same attributes. Although many diseases and afflictions found representation in the pantheon of popular Hinduism, Sitala enjoyed prominence as a deity of exceptional potency. If humoured and honoured through prayers, offerings and devotional acts, she could give protection from the disease or modify its effects. Angered or neglected, however, her wrath took the form of the violent fever that raged through her victims' bodies and resulted in lasting disfigurement or death. Since Sitala was understood to be intrinsically the 'Cool One', she was offered cooling foods and her victims were plied with cold drinks and balms. A patient who died of smallpox was not cremated – the customary practice among many castes in India – for fear of scorching the goddess and further provoking her.[18]

Because the disease followed so familiar a cycle, annual ceremonies were held in the diety's honour in many parts of eastern and northern India during the spring (and smallpox) season. At this time, too, there were Sitala fairs and pilgrimages (especially by women and children) to major shrines to the goddess (such as at Gurgaon, southwest of Delhi).[19]

For most Hindus (and indeed for the many Muslims who shared this aspect of folk culture with Hindus) belief in Sitala and Mariyamma was an integral part of their wider understanding of disease and of benevolent and malevolent forces. As the 'Cool One', Sitala's worship embodied popular beliefs in the antithetical concepts of cooling and heating in ritual and diet. Some of these ideas were not far removed from notions of disease that had been common in Europe in earlier centuries. But to nineteenth-century British doctors, missionaries and administrators such beliefs were rank superstition, evidence only of Indian apathy and ignorance. The duality of the smallpox goddess (protector as well as persecutor) was lost to them. She appeared only as a demon, part of the dark side of Hinduism which, along with *sati, thugi,* and female infanticide, Europeans found deeply repugnant.[20] From a position of such hostility and contempt, the British were ill-placed to understand the tenacity with which Indians clung to their faith in Sitala and hence one of the reasons for the popular antipathy to godless vaccination.

Variolation

If familiarity with a dreaded disease prompted its ritualisation, it also encouraged attempts at medical control. Smallpox was uniquely favourable for this purpose, producing variolous matter from skin eruptions and scabs that could be transferred and absorbed by the recipient through subcutaneous injection, through swallowing, or by inhaling the powdered crusts. The virus itself remained active for at least a year in carefully preserved crusts and, if effectively inoculated, conferred life-long immunity. Transmission required no complex vector relationships and a basic understanding of how the disease passed from one individual to another did not have to await the scientific discoveries of the late nineteenth century. For these reasons the practice of variolation or smallpox inoculation may have developed independently in different parts of Eurasia and Africa rather than being diffused from a single source as is generally assumed. In India it appears to have been long established in the east, in Bengal especially, while in the west, particularly in Sind, its introduction was sometimes attributed to the

Muslim invasions.[21] In the nineteenth century variolation was widely practised in Bengal, Bihar and the eastern half of the North-Western Provinces (today's Uttar Pradesh), but seems to have been uncommon west of Allahabad. It was to be found in parts of the Himalayan region and the Punjab hills, further west in Sind, Gujarat, and Maharashtra, and as far south as Goa (where it was practised by the Portuguese clergy). In Dravidian south India, in the area where Mariyamma replaced Sitala, inoculation, though not unknown, appears to have been far less common. As late as 1801, five years after Jenner's discovery of the prophylactic effects of cowpox, the British in the Madras Presidency were still trying to persuade Indians to adopt inoculation.[22]

As practised in India, variolation had a number of distinctive features. Firstly, it was seen to be sanctioned by religion. Although some Hindus relied upon worship of Sitala alone, for many inoculation was itself a religious ritual. In Bengal it was commonly performed by Brahmins (India's leading ritual specialists) and accompanied by songs and prayers invoking the protective benevolence of the goddess. Further offerings were made to Sitala on the child's recovery from the ordeal of immunisation.[23] Secondly, variolation had its own special practitioners, known as *tikadars* or 'mark-makers' in eastern India. According to J. Z. Holwell's account of variolation in Bengal, published in 1767, the most celebrated of these came from Banaras, Allahabad and Vrindaban.[24] But by the mid-nineteenth century many other castes were also involved, including Malis (a caste of gardeners and agriculturalists) and Sindurias (vermillion-sellers) in northern India and Napits (barbers) in Dhaka (Dacca).[25] Thirdly, variolation was a form of medical treatment sought after and paid for by the people themselves: unlike vaccination, it was not dependent upon state patronage and intervention. Individual *tikadars* had long-standing relations with client villages which they visited every year or two, inoculating large numbers of children at a time.[26]

In a situation where smallpox was almost universal, variolation was practised on a scale the British were unable to match until late in the nineteenth century. In 1871 there may have been twenty times as many variolators as vaccinators in northern Bengal. In 1873 it was reckoned that in one district of Orissa alone a hundred *tikadars* were at work, carrying out 25,000 inoculations in a single season.[27] A 'vaccine census' conducted by the Government of Bengal in 1872–3 revealed that out of 113,015 people examined, 57 per cent had been inoculated, 15.35 per cent had survived an attack of smallpox and so had acquired natural immunity, 10.42 per cent remained unprotected, but only 17.23 per cent had been vaccinated.[28] Other estimates placed the proportion inoculated even higher – at 70 per cent or more of the population of mid-century Bengal.[29] Variolation was certainly not so widespread elsewhere in India, but the figures give some indication of the size of the task that colonial medicine faced in trying to oust an indigenous rival.

The efficacy of variolation has been a matter of some dispute in recent years. Peter Razzell has argued that in eighteenth-century Britain variolation was employed on a sufficiently large scale and with enough care to check smallpox mortality and cause a downturn in the overall death rate.[30] Conventional medical opinion, now as in the nineteenth century, is highly sceptical of such claims and maintains that variolation is doubly dangerous. Inoculating with live smallpox virus exposes patients to the risk of a severe, possibly fatal, attack. In addition, the disease thus transmitted remains as virulent as that contracted in the normal way and is equally capable of spreading smallpox in epidemic form.[31]

In his description of variolation in Bengal, Holwell detailed the careful procedures followed by the *tikadars* and suggested that they were fully aware of the contagious nature of the disease. The *tikadars*, he said, used variolous matter collected the previous year: 'they never inoculated with fresh matter, nor with matter from the disease caught in the natural way, however distinct and mild the species'.[32] This implies that they deliberately propagated an attenuated form of the virus in order to induce a moderate reaction. Holwell claimed that inoculation seldom resulted in the appearance of more than two hundred pustules and sometimes produced as few as fifty. He stressed that variolation did not give rise to epidemics 'as is commonly imagined in Europe'.[33]

After 1802, however, with the introduction of vaccination into India, European physicians took a far more critical view of variolation. John Shoolbred, Bengal's second Superintendent-General of Vaccination, reported Brahmin *tikadars* as admitting to one death in every two hundred clients inoculated, which he compared to a figure of one fatality in three hundred cases in Europe. But, without offering any evidence for his assertion, Shoolbred claimed that the practice was 'certainly much less favourable here than in Europe' and probably caused the death of one in every sixty or seventy of those inoculated.[34] Such was the intensity of British hostility that in 1831, W. Cameron, the Superintendent-General of the day, dubbed variolation a 'murderous trade' and called its suppression 'indispensable to the interests of humanity'.[35]

But British medical officers in India were not entirely unanimous on this point, though there was never any doubt in their minds that vaccination was a superior and a safer practice. Some felt, however, that it would be reckless to ban variolation before vaccination was freely available. T. E. Charles, Bengal's Superintendent-General of Vaccination in 1869, believed that prohibiting variolation would 'constitute a great hardship' to the people unless vaccination could be provided as an 'efficient substitute'. Like J. Wise, Civil Surgeon at Dhaka, Charles doubted whether variolation caused anything like the number of deaths attributed to it by current medical opinion in Britain. Both placed the likely mortality at around one per cent and were sceptical, too, of the view that variolation often sparked off epidemics.[36] Charles went so far as to suggest to the Government of Bengal that variolators should be allowed to continue their work under licence in areas where vaccination was not yet available or widely accepted. His proposal was rejected as giving encouragement to an undesirable practice. The most the government would permit was the recruitment and training of *tikadars* as vaccinators.[37]

Vaccination

The arrival of vaccination marked a new and critical stage in the development of western medicine in India. Hitherto, European practitioners had confined themselves almost exclusively to ministering to the needs of their own community and to the British and Indian soldiers employed by the East India Company. Not only had there been no serious attempt to take medicine to the masses: there existed a profound ignorance about the diseases prevalent in India and the state of health of the bulk of the population. Vaccination was introduced into India at a momentous time. As a result of the rapid expansion of British dominion in South Asia, India's new rulers were beginning to appreciate a need for a more detailed knowledge of the society and the country over which they governed. This included greater knowledge of the causes of mortality and the nature of India's disease environment, factors likely to have a direct bearing on the economic life and even the political security of the new regime. At a time when western medicine could offer few cures or prophylactics, smallpox stood almost alone as a 'preventible disease'. Without sophisticated medical knowledge and at seemingly little expense, smallpox could, it was hoped, be conquered. More could be achieved by vaccination, it was sometimes said, than by any other known sanitary or medical measure.[38]

An appreciative European community, quick to send Jenner £7,000 in thanks for its own delivery from smallpox, confidently anticipated that Indians would take up with 'equal gratitude' a discovery which Europe had already found to confer 'such inestimable benefits'.[39] There was an ill-informed expectation, too, that Hindus, with their famed reverence for the cow and its products, would seize 'with the greatest ardour' this latest bovine boon to man.[40] There were also more practical considerations in view. For a regime but recently established by force of arms and with the struggle against the Marathas still unconcluded, vaccination offered a welcome opportunity to win 'good will from the people' and give 'fresh proof' of Britain's 'humane and benevolent' intentions.[41] In approving expenditure on vaccination in 1805, Lord Bentinck, Governor of Madras, declared himself 'happy in the reflection that no expense was ever made for objects of greater individual happiness or of public advantage'. But he added, more pragmatically, that in a country where the state derived so great a share of its income from the land 'every life saved is additional revenue and an increase to the population and to the prosperity of the Company's territories in an incalculable ratio'.[42]

But expectations of the ready and appreciative acceptance of vaccination were soon dashed. Indians from the outset proved reluctant to submit to vaccination or take up the practice for themselves. Some, as in the villages of Madras, suspecting the government of a 'sinister intention', gathered in crowds to drive away the vaccinators sent to 'diffuse the benefits of vaccination among them'.[43] Such a negative response confirmed many Europeans in an unfavourable view of Indians. Shoolbred in Bengal in 1804 called Hindus 'naturally averse to all innovation' and denounced the labouring classes as 'stupid and insensible' for failing to recognise vaccination's 'inestimable value'.[44] Duncan Stewart, Superintendent-General of Vaccination for the province in the early 1840s, likewise blamed Hindu ingratitude and ignorance, especially 'the trammels of a degrading religion, by which their thoughts are chained, their reasoning faculties hoodwinked and their mutual affections thwarted'. Even 'the most simple, obvious and unquestionable temporal advantage' was, he claimed, unacceptable to Hindus if it entailed 'the slightest deviation from ancient usage'.[45] Such sentiments persisted well into the second half of the century. In 1878, for instance, the North-Western Provinces' Sanitary Commissioner attributed the limited impact of vaccination to the 'natural apathy of the people, their disinclination to accept a new thing, and their unreasonable religious beliefs or caste prejudices'.[46]

Opinions such as these show the ease and frequency with which racial and cultural antipathy clouded British medical and administrative judgement. That vaccination also encountered considerable opposition in Britain was generally ignored: Indians' religion, social practices and customs were instead singled out for blame. In fact, although cultural resistance was undoubtedly an important contributor to vaccination's slow progress in India, it was only one of the inhibiting factors.

Despite the claims often made for the simplicity and effectiveness of vaccination, many technical difficulties stood in the way of its success in India. Commentators who contrast variolation with vaccination are apt to forget how crude and ineffective the latter often was, during the early nineteenth century especially. In India there was, first of all, a problem of supply. Cowpox was rare, possibly unknown, in the country, and until the 1890s much of the vaccine was imported from Britain. The first vaccine reached India in June 1802 through a relay of children vaccinated from arm to arm from Baghdad to Bombay.[47] Subsequently, vaccine crusts or sealed tubes of lymph were sent by sea or brought overland from Britain: India's medical dependency thus replicated its political and economic ties. By the time the lymph came to be used, however, it was often inert, and this was one reason for the high rate of unsuccessful vaccinations in India.[48] Once established, the vaccine was maintained (as in Britain) by the arm-to-arm method. But here, too, there were difficulties. The vaccine was often 'lost' in transmission and during the wet and humid monsoon months vaccination could be ineffective or produced 'foul, sloughing sores'. In consequence, in northern and eastern India the 'vaccination season' was confined to the cooler, drier months between September and March.[49]

For as long as vaccination relied on imported lymph and the arm-to-arm process the scale of operations in India was very limited. In Bombay, the province where vaccination was most enthusiastically pursued, there were only 446,000 vaccinations between 1846 and 1850, with a further 849,000 between 1851 and 1855.[50] From the middle of the century, however, significant advances were made. In the North-Western Provinces depots were established in the hills of Kumaon to collect vaccine crusts and lymph to supply to the plains: some 20,000 crusts were despatched in 1867–8 alone.[51] In the 1850s the Bombay Vaccination Department began experimenting with the production of calf lymph, though it was twenty years before this technique was sufficiently reliable for general use. Arm-to-arm vaccination persisted in parts of Bengal until the First World War, but by that date calf lymph, preserved with glycerine, was being produced in sufficient quantity to end dependence on imported supplies. The Vaccine Institute at Belgaum was manufacturing 600,000 doses of calf vaccine a year by 1911.[52]

As a result of these changes, the scale of vaccination could be substantially increased in the late nineteenth century. From 4.5 million operations a year in the late 1870s, the total for British India rose to 6.5 million a decade later, and touched 9 million in the early years of the twentieth century.[53] There were important advances in technique, too: the lancet was replaced in the 1870s by the vaccinating needle, and fewer punctures were made. This reduced the inconvenience to the labouring classes and the risk of infection. By 1900 vaccination was a far more efficient and reliable operation that it had been thirty or forty years earlier.

The persistence of the arm-to-arm method of vaccination also highlights one of the reasons for vaccination's early unpopularity. Unlike variolation, where old crusts were used (sanctified with a sprinkling of Ganges water), vaccination transferred body fluids directly from one individual to another. For most Hindus this was ritually very polluting, especially since low-caste or untouchable children were usually the only vaccinifers: higher caste parents went to great trouble to ensure that their children were not used in this way.[54] The extraction of lymph from a child's arm could be alarmingly painful. According to Surgeon-Captain H. J. Dyson, Sanitary Commissioner for Bengal in 1893:

> The child, attended by its weeping mother, is taken round the town or village, and sometimes from one village to another, and after all the lymph has been extracted from the vesicles on its arms, it is a common practice for the vaccinators to squeeze the inflammed base of the vaccine pustules further in order to obtain serum for more vaccinations.

In his experience, the 'agony caused to the child was often intense'. Vaccination could result in long periods of suffering caused by 'severe and deep ulcers', and sometimes there were fatal complications. Dyson urged that calf lymph should replace arm-to-arm vaccination as quickly as possible, even though the expense was considerably greater.[55]

Substituting calf lymph, however, created problems of its own. Many Hindus believed that taking lymph from calves involved the animals in unacceptable suffering. Opposition to the practice was particularly strong in western India in the 1870s and 1880s: some municipalities refused to grant funds for the purpose and individual contractors were subjected to such pressure that they declined to supply heifers for vaccination purposes.[56] With time, however, opposition died away and many Indians clearly preferred the use of calf vaccine to the old arm-to-arm method. There was some revival of opposition during the Non-Co-operation Movement in the early 1920s, and Gandhi expressed his personal distaste for vaccination which he described as a 'filthy process' and 'little short of taking beef'.[57] But Gandhi's views on this matter did not command much public support and by the 1930s vaccination had won a wide degree of acceptance in India.

Vaccination was disliked for other reasons, too. Unlike variolation, usually performed on children over five, vaccination was primarily directed at infants under one year old, an age at which many mothers felt them to be too young for such an operation.[58] The mildness of the reaction produced by vaccination – one of its virtues in British eyes – was often taken as an indication of its ineffectiveness compared to inoculation. Scepticism was increased by the high failure rate from vaccination compared to the lifelong immunity acquired through variolation.[59] This was also an obstacle to revaccination: another was that it involved exposing girls of post-pubertal age to the touch of a male vaccinator.[60]

But one of the greatest objections to vaccination was its secularity. There was no dietary or ritual preparation as in variolation; no invocation of Sitala; no priestly ministrations to provide reassurance during and after the operation. Such an 'irreligious' act was thought to be offensive to the goddess and was certainly out of keeping with the religious conceptualisation of disease and medicine among Hindus and Muslims alike.[61] There was, however, some room for compromise. Despite the disapproval of their superintendents, some Indian vaccinators (especially those who had formerly been *tikadars*) diluted the raw secularity of their work with a few Sitala prayers and rituals. Parents also took the initiative, delaying vaccination until an auspicious day or hour and employing priests to seek Sitala's blessing.[62] In many respects rivals, variolation and vaccination were at least comparable forms of medical intervention: vaccination could be offered as a superior form of an existing prophylaxis. Resistance to it was often greatest among tribal communities with no prior experience of variolation or among religious sects, like the Faraizis, Muslim fundamentalists of eastern Bengal, for whom variolation and vaccination were equally unacceptable forms of interference with 'God's will'.[63]

In striking contrast with the colonial image of western medicine as the benevolent gift of a superior civilisation, vaccination aroused in many Indians a deep suspicion of the nature and purposes of British rule. Why, it was wondered, were the British so keen to put their mark (*tika*) upon the people? The explanations provided by popular rumour perceived a basic malevolence or self-interest on the part of the British at Indians' expense. Vaccination was said to be a deliberate attempt to violate caste and religion and so make converts to Christianity. Those marked by vaccination would later die in agony or be sacrificed to ensure the successful completion of a bridge or railway embankment. Vaccination was feared as the prelude to new taxation or forced labour. One of the commonest beliefs was that the British were searching for a child with white blood or milk in his veins: this would be the saviour (the Mahdi of the Muslims) who would drive out the foreigners unless first caught and destroyed.[64] To British medical officers and administrators such tales were further evidence of Indian ingratitude and ignorance. Viewed more sympatheticallly, however, they testify to a deep distrust of British rule and show how readily state medical intervention was identified with other coercive and alien aspects of the colonial regime.

A question of agency

Confident that vaccination would gain rapid acceptance in India, the British at first gave little thought to the need for a permanent vaccination agency. It was assumed that once the practice became popular Indians would take it up for themselves at minimal cost to the state. It was not long, however, before this early optimism evaporated and the state's financial commitment to vaccination was viewed with growing concern. As early as 1808 the Government of India was advising caution over expenditure on vaccination and futher directives in 1811 urged reductions as soon as the practice became general among the Indian population. In 1829 the Government of Bengal decided that the expense of running thirty vaccination centres was unjustified by the results and all but six were abolished.[65]

Bombay, however, developed a more ambitious vaccination programme. Under the direction of the Governor, Lord Elphinstone, a scheme was devised in 1827 to carry vaccination to the rural population. The province was divided into circles, each with its own team of itinerant vaccinators. These were to visit each village at least once a year and provide free vaccination to as many children as possible. The vaccinators were to be Indians, but, following an administrative pattern common in colonial India, they were placed under European inspectors, who were to examine their returns and check on their work. The Bombay system was said to have two 'great merits': 'it brought vaccination to the doors of the people – too lazy, too poor, or too ignorant to seek it', and 'it ensured the examination by the European medical officer of every case attended upon'.[66] Seen to be successful in Bombay, the scheme was introduced into several other provinces (though not Bengal) in the 1850s and 1860s.

But the Bombay system had its limitations. There were frequent reports of vaccinators submitting false returns, exaggerating the number of vaccinations actually performed, or being too illiterate to fill in the forms correctly. Low-caste vaccinators were thought to command little public respect, and in general much was seen to rest upon a rather unreliable subordinate agency. In the words of the Madras Sanitary Commissioner in 1884, 'nothing tends more to injure the cause of vaccination than incompetent and untrustworthy agency'.[67]

The creation of a special vaccination staff and the setting up of provincial vaccination departments were not in themselves sufficient, therefore, to ensure the success of vaccination. In Bengal, where the challenge from variolation was strongest, the government adopted a series of expedients to try to supplant the rival practice. Soon after vaccination was first introduced into the province attempts were made to recruit some of the leading *tikadars* as government vaccinators and persuade Brahmin pandits to issue public declarations that there was nothing in the Hindu *sastras* or sacred texts that prohibited vaccination or made variolation a religious duty.[68] This ploy had little effect, however, and in Calcutta, the principal seat of British power in India, the number of variolators appears actually to have increased during the early nineteenth century.[69]

Further attempts at co-opting variolators were made in Bengal and the North-Western Provinces in the 1870s. In 1873 Bengal alone counted 472 ex-*tikadars* among its vaccinators and five years later there were nearly 1,000 of them. It was hoped that by allowing them to charge for their services vaccination would in time become independent of state subsidy.[70] But the scheme met with little success. Villagers would not pay for a vaccination they did not want and vaccinators could collect their fees only with difficulty. In the past variolators had earned substantial sums – one in Banaras division boasted of receiving Rs 80 to 90 a month – and few were willing to forgo the profit and prestige of a *tikadar* to become a despised state vaccinator on Rs 10 to 18 a month. In fact, a number of ex-variolators quickly reverted to their former calling.[71] European medical officers also had strong prejudices against recruiting such men, seeing them (the lower caste variolators especially) to be shabby, untrustworthy and an offence to their own professionalism.[72]

One alternative strategy was to look beyond the formal vaccination agency to leading Indians in the hope that these might use their influence and authority to encourage vaccination among their families, followers and dependents. This was a strategy much favoured in the North-Western Provinces where British power rested heavily upon the 'chiefs and landlords of the people'. Among those whose 'wisdom and philanthropy' were successfully invoked in the late nineteenth century were the rajas of Banaras, Balrampur and Tehri.[73] In western India, however, the strategy brought less success and it was only with difficulty that the rulers of princely states could be persuaded to allow vaccinators to operate in their territories.[74] In the cities, government servants, newspaper editors, lawyers and educationalists were also enrolled in the cause of vaccination; but some of India's most influential urban residents, the Marwari and Bania merchants, traders and moneylenders, were among the most resolute opponents of vaccination – partly from religious scruple, but also because they were generally resistant to most westernising influences.[75]

Attempts to shift a large share of the financial burden and administrative responsibility for vaccination onto the newly created municipal and local boards was also no more than a qualified success. Indian councillors were often personally unenthusiastic about vaccination and reluctant to divert scarce funds to so unpopular a cause. Even when compulsory vaccination was introduced by law many municipalities in practice dragged their feet and failed to perform the number of vaccinations required.[76]

Frustration at the slow progress of vaccination, at continuing high levels of smallpox mortality, and the persistence of variolation, produced strong pressure from the medical profession for legislative action. The first move in this direction – Lord Wellesley's ban on variolation in Calcutta in 1804 – was so ineffectual that it was soon abandoned, and for several decades no further moves were made. Fifty years after Wellesley, another Governor-General, Lord Dalhousie, declared that it was as impossible to prohibit variolation as it was to 'make the monsoon penal'.[77] In 1872 Sir John Strachey of the Viceroy's Council opposed a draft vaccination bill prepared by the Bombay government on the grounds that any attempt to impose vaccination by force would provoke resistance and make it even more unpopular than at present. He argued that the 'prejudices of the people' could only be overcome by gradual persuasion and example.[78] The virtues of 'patience and time' were again urged on the Bombay government when it submitted a revised bill five years later.[79]

But, for all the Government of India's prevarication, the provincial administrations were coming to see the need for some form of legislation. Recent enactments in Britain, outlawing variolation and making vaccination compulsory, provided influential precedents. In 1865 variolation was banned in Calcutta and its suburbs, and in 1866 the prohibition was extended to surrounding villages as well.[80] Faced with repeated epidemics, and confident that it now had sufficient vaccine for the purpose, in 1877 the Government of Bombay finally passed its own Vaccination Act. This made vaccination compulsory within the city of Bombay for all infants under six months old and for all children under fourteen brought into the city from outside on penalty of six months' imprisonment or Rs. 1,000 fine for the parent or guardian. Inoculation was prohibited and no recently inoculated person was to enter the city.[81] A similar act was passed for Karachi in 1879, and the Bombay legislation became the basis for the Government of India's own Vaccination Act in 1880.

The dramatic decline in the number of deaths due to smallpox in Bombay and Karachi following the introduction of compulsory vaccination provided an argument for the further extension of legal measures. The voluntary system had been 'ineffectual', the Bombay government reasoned, not so much because of religious objections as from public 'indifference, indolence or ignorance'.[82] But the colonial authorities remained wary. Quite apart from financial considerations, the administration (especially in the North-Western Provinces and Punjab) remained nervous of a public backlash against coercive medical intervention. The mere rumour of compulsory vaccination was enough to set off a scare and threaten disturbances in Delhi in 1870–71.[83] The intensity of the public reaction against compulsory anti-plague measures (again mostly in northern India) in 1898–1900 further hinted at the political risks medical interventionism might entail for an alien goverment.[84] In consequence the Government of India allowed only a gradual extension of the 1880 Vaccination Act: by 1906 it had been introduced in 441 towns and cantonments, representing only seven per cent of British India's total population. Very few small towns and rural areas were included before the 1930s. Even in 1950, three years after India's independence, vaccination was compulsory in no more than 732 of the country's 842 municipalities and barely half of its 408,000 villages.[85]

The Vaccination Act was also notoriously difficult to enforce. Registration of births, begun in the 1870s, remained so defective that vaccination staff had no clear idea of the number of infants requiring vaccination. In major cities like Bombay there was the further complication of high rates of immigration from the countryside with many babies and children arriving unvaccinated and unregistered. Prosecutions were few, partly from lack of interest by the police, magistracy and municipal authorities. In some municipalities in the 1880s and 1890s the Vaccination Act was frankly admitted to be a 'dead letter'.[86]

As a result, upwards of twenty per cent of infants even in the best vaccinated urban areas escaped vaccination. Although immunisation significantly reduced the number of susceptibles, there remained a substantial pool of children and adults among whom smallpox could continue to circulate. Epidemics were becoming less frequent in the early twentieth century, but they numbered an increasing percentage of adults among their victims.[87] The nineteenth-century assumption that vaccination made smallpox a 'preventible disease' was thus only partly valid. The need also to isolate smallpox cases and their contacts was urged from time to time during the century, but was always rejected as entailing too great an interference in the lives of the people and requiring an army of medical subordinates for its enforcement.[88] Again, the experience of the early plague years, 1896–1900, showed the practical and political snares such measures were likely to encounter. In consequence, smallpox was not even made a notifiable disease in colonial India, and it was not until the international smallpox eradication campaign of the 1960s and 1970s that the disease was finally tackled in a sufficiently comprehensive way to ensure its final extinction in India.

Conclusion

Medical intervention against smallpox in nineteenth-century India was only partly constrained by a lack of appropriate epidemiological knowledge and immunisation technology. Smallpox was a disease as familiar to Europe as to South Asia; its basic mode of transmission was well understood; and there existed in vaccination an at least potentially effective prophylaxis. To some extent the problems vaccination encountered in India mirrored European experience – the reluctance of people to seek vaccination (except during epidemics), the low level of immunity conferred (until the introduction of revaccination and improved vaccine preservation methods), and the difficulty of creating a suitable mass immunisation agency. But in many respects the history of smallpox and vaccination in India is expressive of a colonial situation in which the administration was culturally and politically remote from the lives of its subjects.

Belief in a smallpox deity provided an alternative, religious, explanation for the incidence of the disease and prescribed ritual observances that ran counter to western medical secularism. In variolation, too, vaccination found a formidable rival, sustained by a specialised agency of its own. It enjoyed the confidence of the people and (until late in the nineteenth century) was more readily available in many parts of the country than state vaccination. Disdainful of indigenous belief and folk practice, the British medical establishment was as loath to compromise with Sitala as it was with variolation. But while there could be no question of outlawing disease deities, the British saw the supplanting of variolation as essential to the success of their own medical system. As far as vaccination was concerned, medical monopoly, not cultural pluralism, was the desired goal. Finding persuasion, co-option, and the enlistment of leading Indians, inadequate for the purpose, the colonial authorities eventually turned to legislation to ban variolation and hasten public acceptance of vaccination. An exotic, without root on Indian soil, vaccination long remained closely identified with foreign rule, attracting suspicions and fears that ranged far beyond doubts about its medical efficacy. The negative character of British attitudes to Sitala and variolation was thus matched by Indian antipathy to vaccination and the coercive, unheeding system of colonialism it was taken to represent.

To perhaps a greater degree than in Britain, vaccination in India was inhibited by technical difficulties – there were problems of climate, for example, and of obtaining sufficient pure lymph. But it was constrained, too, by the nature of the colonial regime itself. Disposed to see the health of its European subjects and servants as a first priority, the colonial state was reluctant to make the financial and administrative commitment necessary for an effective assault on smallpox. The sheer size and expense of such an undertaking was always a deterrent. But there was an inhibiting ambivalence in British attitudes as well. Vaccination was welcomed as a demonstration of the superiority of West over East, science over superstition. And yet, from an abiding sense of policial insecurity, heightened by the Mutiny and Rebellion of 1857–8 and by rumbling discontent over other forms of medical intervention, the state shied away from a vaccination programme that might provoke resistance and revolt. A fear of the consequences of compulsion was thus an important check on the state and on the medical profession's interventionist ambitions. It encouraged greater reliance, in this field of colonial activity as in many others, on persuasion, on Indian intermediaries, and upon a gradualist approach to the prospect of social change.

Notes

Earlier versions of this chapter were presented to the Society for the Social History of Medicine conference at Aston University in April 1986 and at the History of Medicine seminar at University College, London, in November 1986. I am grateful to all those who commented on the paper on these occasions, and also to Paul Greenough for his valuable criticisms.

1 *Annual Report upon Vaccination in the North-Western Provinces, 1866–7* (hereafter cited as *NWP VR, 1866–7*), p. 4; T. E. Charles, *Popular Information on Smallpox, Inoculation and Vaccination,* Calcutta, 1870, p. 1; S. P. James, *Smallpox and Vaccination in British India,* Calcutta, 1909, p. 1.
2 James, *Smallpox,* p. 50.
3 David Arnold, 'Touching the body: perspectives on the Indian plague, 1896–1900', in Ranajit Guha (ed.), *Subaltern Studies,* V, Delhi, 1987, pp. 55-90.
4 It has sometimes been argued that smallpox vaccination was responsible for a massive population increase in the Dutch colony of Java during the nineteenth century. Scholars are now sceptical both that such a large increase actually occurred and that vaccination was sufficiently widespread and effective before the late nineteenth century to have had much demographic effect. See Bram Peper, 'Population growth in Java in the nineteenth century: a new interpretation', *Population Studies,* XXIV, 1970, pp. 71-84. The parallels with India seem close.
5 Ralph W. Nicholas, 'The goddess Sitala and epidemic smallpox in Bengal', *Journal of Asian Studies,* XLI, 1981, pp. 25-6.
6 Nicholas, 'Sitala', pp. 32-4.
7 E.g., *Review of the Madras Famine, 1876–78,* Madras, 1881, p. 150; A. B. Christie, 'Smallpox' in G. Melvyn Howe (ed.), *A World Geography of Human Diseases,* London, 1977, p. 267.
8 Nicholas, 'Sitala', p. 39.
9 Leonard Rogers, *Smallpox and Climate in India,* London, 1926; *Annual Report of the Sanitary Commissioner of the North-Western Provinces, 1886* (hereafter *NWP SCR, 1886*), p. 26.
10 *Report of the Smallpox Commissioners,* Calcutta, 1850, p. 3; *Bengal VR, 1872,* p. 7.
11 Quoted in James, *Smallpox,* p. 49.
12 James, *Smallpox,* pp. 76-7.
13 J. Z. Holwell, *An Account of the Manner of Inoculating for the Smallpox in the East Indies,* London, 1767, p. 4.
14 *Smallpox Commissioners,* pp. 20-2.
15 *Smallpox Commissioners,* p. 24.
16 Deputy Sanitary Commissioner, Central District, to Sanitary Commissioner, Bombay, 17 July 1893, Bombay General, 1, 706, Maharashtra State Archives, Bombay.
17 Assam Vaccination Report, 1881–2, Home (Sanitary), 115, September 1882, National Archives of India, New Delhi (hereafter NAI); *Bengal VR, 1915–16,* p. 2.
18 Nicholas, 'Sitala'; Susan S. Wadley, 'Sitala: the Cool One', *Asian Folklore Studies,* XXXIX, 1980, pp. 33-62; Lawrence A. Babb, *The Divine Hierarchy: Popular Hinduism in Central India,* New York, 1975, pp. 126-32.
19 William Crooke, *The Popular Religion and Folklore of Northern India,* 1, 1896, reprinted Delhi, 1968, p. 126; *NWP SCR, 1881,* p. 25.
20 *Missionary Register for 1836,* London, 1836, p. 465; R. Caldwell, 'On demonolatry in southern India', *Journal of the Anthropological Society of Bombay,* 1, 1887, pp. 91-105.
21 *Bombay VR, 1874–5,* p. 30.
22 Madras Board of Revenue Proceedings, 20 January 1801, Board's Collections, F/4/96/1953, India Office Records, London (IOR).
23 *NWP VR, 1872–3,* p. 31.
24 Holwell, *Account,* p. 8.
25 *NWP VR, 1869–70,* pp. 20-3; *Bengal VR, 1867–8,* pp. 3-4; *Bengal VR, 1872,* p. 56.
26 *NWP VR, 1872–3,* p. 31; Holwell, *Account,* pp. 18-20.
27 *Bengal VR, 1871,* p. 14; Home (Public), 156, March 1873, NAI.
28 *Bengal VR, 1873,* pp. 100-1.
29 *Smallpox Commissioners,* p. 28; James, *Smallpox,* p. 6. Variolation declined sharply in the late nineteenth century but lingered on in some remoter areas well into the following century, e.g. in Sind: *Bombay VR, 1920–1,* p. 3.

30 Peter Razzell, *The Conquest of Smallpox: The Impact of Inoculation on Smallpox Mortality in Eighteenth Century Britain*, Firle, 1977; cf., Paul R. Greenough, 'Variolation and vaccination in South Asia, c. 1700–1865: a preliminary note', *Social Science and Medicine*, XIV, 1980, pp. 345-7.
31 Thomas McKeown, *The Modern Rise of Population*, London, 1976, pp. 11-12, 107-9.
32 Holwell, *Account*, p. 17.
33 Holwell, *Account*, pp. 4, 30.
34 John Shoolbred, *Report on the Progress of Vaccine Inoculation in Bengal, 1802–3*, Calcutta, 1804, pp. 27-8.
35 *Smallpox Commissioners*, p. 54.
36 T. E. Charles, 'Report on the necessity for regulating the practice of smallpox inoculation in Bengal', in *Bengal VR, 1869*, pp. 1-11; J. Wise to Commissioner, Dhaka Division, 14 September 1871, Home (Public), 366, February 1872, NAI.
37 *Bengal VR, 1871*, p. v.
38 *NWP VR, 1873–4*, p. 13; *NWP SCR, 1886*, pp. 26-7.
39 James, *Smallpox*, p. 20; Madras Public Consultations, 19 January 1803, Board's Collections, F/4/153/2613, IOR.
40 Shoolbred, *Report*, p. 82.
41 John Z. Bowers, 'The odyssey of smallpox vaccination', *Bulletin of the History of Medicine*, LV, 1981, p. 24; Archibald Seton, Agent, to Magistrate, Bareilly, 7 June 1805, Bengal Public Consultations, 4 October 1805, Board's Collections, F/4/198/4452, IOR.
42 Minute, 18 June 1805, Board's Collections, F/14/201/4544, IOR.
43 A. McKenzie, Superintendent-General of Vaccine Inoculation, to Secretary, Madras, 5 September 1806, Judicial Proceedings, 31 October 1806, Board's Collections, F/4/268/5891, IOR.
44 Shoolbred, *Report*, pp. 20, 26.
45 Duncan Stewart, *Report on Smallpox in Calcutta, 1833–34, 1837–38, 1843–44*, Calcutta, 1844, p. 9.
46 *NWP SCR, 1878*, p. 30.
47 Shoolbred, *Report*, pp. 2-4.
48 James, *Smallpox*, p. 37; *Bombay VR, 1867*, p. xxi.
49 *Smallpox Commissioners*, pp. 50-51; *NWP SCR, 1876*, p. 28; *NWP VR, 1895–96*, p. 14.
50 *Report on Measures adopted for Sanitary Improvements in India during the year 1868*, London, 1869, p. 137. At this date vaccination reached only an estimated 1.5 per cent of the population in the Bombay Presidency.
51 James, *Smallpox*, pp. 37-8.
52 *Bombay VR, 1908–11; Bengal VR, 1915–16*, p. 3.
53 James, *Smallpox*, p. 76.
54 *Bengal VR, 1867–8*, p. 13; *NWP VR, 1869–70*, p. 2; *Bengal VR, 1896–9*, p. 10.
55 H. J. Dyson to Secretary, Bengal, 30 June 1893, Bengal, Municipal (Sanitation), 3, July 1894, West Bengal State Archives, Calcutta (WBSA).
56 *Bombay VR, 1870–71*, p. 89; *Bombay VR, 1874–5*, p. 19; *Bombay VR, 1890–91*, p. 5.
57 D. G. Tendulkar, *Mahatma: Life of Mohandas Karamchand Gandhi*, III, Delhi, 1961, p. 4.
58 'The prejudice in Hindustan against doing anything to or even looking at young children is a great obstacle to successful vaccination': Oudh (Awadh) Vaccination Report, 1872–3, Home (Public), 495, July 1873, NAI.
59 *Smallpox Commissioners*, pp. lxviii, lxxii; *Bombay VR, 1867*, p. 10; *NWP VR, 1872–3*, p. 29.
60 *Bombay VR, 1905–6*, p. 1.
61 A. Christison, *Report on the Vaccine Operations in the Agra Division, 1858–59*, (no publication data), p. 9.
62 Medical, 75, February 1867, WBSA; *Bengal VR, 1872*, p. 45; *NWP VR, 1872–3*, p. 32.
63 *Bengal VR, 1877*, p. 7; *Bengal VR, 1873*, p. 18; *Bengal VR, 1878*, p. 25; *Bengal VR, 1893–6*, pp. xxiv-xxviii.

64 *Bengal VR, 1867–8,* p. 2; *Bengal VR, 1869,* pp. xix, xliv; *Bengal VR, 1877,* p. 10; *Bengal VR, , 1893–6,* p. xxvi; *Bombay VR, 1858–9,* p. 25; *Bombay VR, 1865,* p. 2; *NWP VR, 1870–1,* p. 11; *NWP VR, 1873–4,* p. 21.
65 *Bengal VR, 1867–8,* p. 5; Public to Bengal, 6 April 1808, Board's Collections, F/4/297/6889; Public to Bengal, 3 September 1813, Board's Collections, F/4/446/10749, IOR.
66 James, *Smallpox,* p. 21.
67 *Madras SCR, 1884,* p. 113.
68 Board's Collections, F/4/186/3906, IOR; *Smallpox Commissioners,* pp. 28-9, xxii; *Bengal VR, 1870,* p. 3.
69 *Smallpox Commissioners,* p. 35.
70 *Bengal VR, 1873,* p. 1; James, *Smallpox,* p. 31.
71 *NWP VR, 1869–70,* p. 23; *NWP VR, 1871–2,* p. 24; *Bengal VR, 1872,* pp. 45-6.
72 *NWP VR, 1872–3,* pp. 13, 32; *Bengal VR, 1872,* p. 21.
73 *NWP VR, 1872–3,* p. 11; *NWP SCR, 1878,* p. 30; *NWP SCR, 1879,* pp. 35, 39.
74 *Bombay VR, 1868,* p. xvii.
75 *Bombay VR, 1867,* p. 19; *NWP VR, 1872–3,* pp. 14, 27; *Bengal VR, 1873,* p. 4; *Administration Report of the Commissioner of Calcutta for 1898–99,* Calcutta, 1899, part 2, pp. 39-40.
76 *Madras VR, 1890–91,* p. 7.
77 James, *Smallpox,* p. 14; *Papers on Vaccination in India,* Calcutta, 1851; Home (Public), 156, March 1873, NAI.
78 Strachey, 3 October 1872, Home (Public), 151-3, notes, November 1872, NAI.
79 *Bombay VR, 1875–6,* p. 1.
80 James, *Smallpox,* p. 14.
81 R. D. Dalal, *Manual of Vaccination for the Bombay Presidency,* Bombay, 1930, part 2, pp. 69-77.
82 Home (Judicial), 89, February 1890, NAI.
83 Home (Public), 246, April 1872, NAI.
84 Arnold, 'Touching the body'.
85 James, *Smallpox,* p. 33; *Statistical Appendices to Annual Report of the Director-General of Health Services, 1950,* Delhi, 1955, p. 53.
86 *Bombay VR, 1895–6,* p. 22; *Madras VR, 1893–4,* p. 5.
87 *Madras VR, 1898–9,* p. 2; James *Smallpox,* p. 100.
88 *Bengal VR, 1869,* p. xiii and p. i of government review.

CHAPTER FOUR

Medicine and racial politics: changing images of the New Zealand Maori in the nineteenth century

Malcolm Nicolson

Throughout the nineteeenth century, virtually all British commentators agreed as to the inherent biological and cultural inferiority of non-European peoples.[1] There was however a considerable diversity of opinion as to the precise nature and degree of that inferiority and the extent to which it could be remedied. As we shall see these were matters of considerable political as well as academic importance. Perceptions of the ability of the indigenous peoples to respond to the challenges posed by contact with European civilisation played a key role in debates over imperial native policy. This essay will argue that the testimony of medical men occupied a central position in this aspect of Victorian polemic and policy-making. It will do this by examining a selection of nineteenth-century medical attitudes toward the Polynesian people of New Zealand, the Maori.

All those interested in the history of European attitudes to the Pacific and its indigenous races are greatly in the debt of Bernard Smith. In his pathfinding study *European Vision in the South Pacific*, Professor Smith documented how, throughout the eighteenth and early nineteenth centuries, portrayals of the lands and peoples of the South Pacific varied as the social basis of European involvement in the region developed.[2] From voyages of exploration to missionary activity, to imperial annexation and large-scale settlement, each form of European interaction with the South Pacific had its own characteristic perceptions of the landscapes and the races encountered. Smith also pointed out that representations of the indigenous peoples varied as artists and authors appealed to different European audiences. Polynesians might be portrayed as Noble, Ignoble or Romantic Savages according to who the artist was and what cultural function his representation was intended to fulfil.

Smith drew his evidence from paintings, engravings, journals and poems. He did not apply his social analysis to the scientific perceptions of the peoples of the South Pacific. Indeed he perceived a tension between, on the one hand, aesthetic and ideological conventions as to how the Polynesians should be portrayed and the demands of empirical scientific investigation, on the other. He saw the ideas of the Noble, Ignoble and Romantic Savage as existing 'despite the objective investigations of scientists, educated missionaries and travellers'.[3] After 1820, Smith argued, the 'dry light of science' withered away the earlier subjective depictions of the peoples of the South Pacific.[4]

It is of course undeniable that the graphic arts achieved considerably greater accuracy in the service of nineteenth-century science. However the present essay argues that the triumph of objectivity in Victorian perceptions of the South Pacific has been overstated. Medical and scientific views of the Maori in the nineteenth century were not wholly or uniquely determined by the objective scrutiny of empirical reality. On the contrary Victorian medical knowledge of the Maori was as thoroughly structured by convention and ideology as the images produced by eighteenth-century artists. Nineteenth-century equivalents of the Noble, Ignoble and Romantic Savage can readily be found. In other words *European Vision in the South Pacific* is a more valuable aid to our understanding of nineteenth-century perceptions of the indigenous peoples of the South Pacific than its author allows.

It will also be argued that nineteenth-century views of the Maori were devised and employed for particular social and political purposes. In the social deployment of images of the Maori lies the full explanation for the lack of agreement among nineteenth-century observers as to the nature and extent of their inferiority. The range of opinion about the Maoris' ability and potential exactly mirrors the diversity of European political involvement in New Zealand. Missionaries, imperial authorities and settlers all constructed their own vision of the Maori. The distinctive characteristics of each image aided the particular social interests of the political grouping for whom it was devised.

The essay will also consider some of the institutions of imperial medicine. It will be argued that the provision of hospitals for the Maori was also undertaken with quite specific social and political purposes in view. Just as different interest groups constructed different images of the Maori, so native hospitals were built for a variety of social reasons. The exact parallel which may be made between the social function of medical knowledge and medical institutions provides strong support for one of the principal conclusions of this essay – namely that medical knowledge of the indigenous peoples of the Empire is best regarded in an instrumental and materialistic manner, as part of the technology of empire, as one of the vast variety of tools with which European historical actors sought to advance their social and material interests in the colonies.[5]

John Savage's Noble Savages

In the late eighteenth and early nineteenth centuries, the Maoris did not get quite as good a press as some of their Polynesian cousins. While the Tahitians were regularly held to be the very ideal of the Noble Savage, the Maoris were perhaps as often portrayed as the ignoble equivalent.[6] This view was founded upon their reputation as ferocious cannibals. The killing and eating of the French navigator Marion de Fresne, together with some of his crew, by Maoris in 1772 and the Rowe massacre in 1773 provided ample evidence in support of this opinion.[7] Such condemnation was not however universal. Even those who were horrified by their cannibalism often found other qualities to admire. Some commentators wholeheartedly commended the Maori on their fine physiques, their military virtues and their relatively advanced social organisation.[8] The earliest nineteenth-century medical account of the Maori embodies this more optimistic perception.

John Savage visited New Zealand in 1806 on the whaler *Ferret*. Suspended from his post as Assistant Surgeon to New South Wales following allegations of professional misconduct, he was on his way back to London to appeal to Earl Fitzwilliam, Lord President of the Council.[9] He seems to have spent several weeks at the Bay of Islands. His description of the Maoris is very positive indeed.

> The natives of New Zealand . . . are of a very superior order, both in point of personal appearance and intellectual endowment . . . The men are . . . well proportioned and exhibit evident marks of great strength. Their countenances are in general open . . . you clearly discover signs of undaunted courage and a resolution not easily shaken.[10]

He has praise for the women too:

> Their features in general are regular and pleasing, with long black hair and dark penetrating eyes . . . I can conceive to a New Zealand lover, their well-formed figures, the interesting cast of their countenance, and the sweet tone of their voice, must render them extremely desirable companions, to sooth his cares, and strew his path through life with flowers.[11]

John Savage never explicitly states that the way of life of the Maori is to be preferred to that of civilised countries. To this extent he stops short of giving full expression to the idea of the Noble Savage.[12] Nevertheless, in his description of New Zealand, he comes very close indeed to emulating the eighteenth-century accounts of Tahiti as an Earthly Paradise peopled by beautiful and virtuous children of Nature.[13]

The Maoris' advantages are not confined to the handsomeness of their countenances or the quality of their physique. In a manner reminiscent of the classic descriptions of Tahiti by Bougainville and Hawkesworth, Savage praises the healthiness of New Zealand: 'That the climate is salubrious cannot be doubted, for neither the appearance or accounts of the natives indicate the prevalence of disease. From this happy state medical practice has hitherto been unknown among them',[4] and of the Maoris' simple way of life: 'The natives have great aversion from spirits, and I do not find that they have any mode of intoxication among them; they are consequently robust cheerful and active, and probably in many instances, live to a great age.'[15]

He dons the cloak of medical authority to endorse the innocent, natural nakedness of the Maori children: 'They are robust, lively and possess in general pleasing countenances; their actions are totally unrestrained by clothing or bandage, which must undoubtedly lay the foundation of their future hardihood and healthy constitution.'[16]

Untutored as they are, the Maori have well-developed moral and religious senses. According to Savage they worship the sun and the moon as deities and believe in a system of rewards and punishments in a future state. They are savages of natural sensibility.[17] They show warm affection for their friends and relatives and they are solicitous as to the welfare of their children. Savage recounts how a canoe carrying women and children to the ship overturned in heavy seas. Each woman contrived to hold onto the hull of the canoe with one hand and onto her child with the other. One of the *Ferret*'s boats was launched and all were rescued. The concern shown by the Maoris on the ship towards those in the water impressed Savage:

> The congratulations on their escape, and their kind and soothing attentions were such as would by no means have disgraced the moral character of the most refined European . . . It was upon this occurrence only that the natives received any strong liquor; I prevailed upon them to take a little wine, which their confidence in me induced them to receive as a medicine to prevent the effects of cold; showing however the greatest solicitude for the health of their children by helping them before they took themselves.[18]

Savage comments elsewhere that the children are 'treated with a great degree of parental affection'.[19]

Savage also gives a favourable picture of Maori society. By his account it is very far from the every-man-for-himself anarchy that some other authors had attributed to primitive peoples.[20] Instead the Maoris have a well-developed civil order which effectively subordinates the individual to the social group:

> In New Zealand as in all uncivilised countries, the passions are the principal guides to the actions of its inhabitants; but in this island I conceive those actions are very much restrained, either by the superintendence and authority of their chiefs or by a natural proneness to affection . . . a great degreee of subordination and affection is observable among them upon all occasions.[21]

Moreover the Maori is portrayed as being, despite appearances and reputation, a peaceable race. Savage makes no mention of the endemic internecine tribal warfare which so dismayed other early commentators.[22] He describes the Maoris trading for axes, adzes and hatchets but he does not mention the trade in weapons nor any exercise or practice of martial skills. He even refers to New Zealand as 'a peaceful isle'.[23] All in all, Savage's description of the Maoris is about as close to the ideal of the Noble Savage as nineteenth-century views of primitive peoples would permit. New Zealand is a mythic unspoilt Eden where Nature is bountiful and Man is innocent and happy:

> Remote in Southern Seas an Island lies,
> Of ample Space, and blessed with Genial skies;
> Where shelter'd still by never-fading groves,
> The friendly Native dwells, and fearless roves;
> Where the tall Forest, and the Plains around,
> And Waters wide, with various wealth abound.[24]

As noted above Savage never claims that the Maoris' lifestyle is to be preferred to that of civilised man. On the other hand he is not convinced that European civilisation promises much benefit to the Maori. On the contrary increased European contact will bring much danger. Following earlier commentators who had foretold the corruption of Tahiti, Savage fears that the earthly paradise of New Zealand is mortally threatened.[25] There is, for instance, already a need for physic where none previously existed: 'I much fear the visits of some European ships have rendered professional assistance necesssary to prevent great numbers of them from falling victims to a most distressing malady.'[26] The Fall is imminent. Venereal disease will be the serpent in the garden:

> Let us for a moment consider its application to New Zealand; a race of people hitherto enjoying a constitution of body remarkably sound and healthy. In a few generations, in all probability, how great will be the change – children of diseased parents, they will grow up a puny race; and, in many instances both miserable and disgusting; in no respect resembling the hardy inhabitants of the island, previously to their unhappy communications with civilised man.[27]

Savage writes in a manner typical of the eighteenth-century travel journal. He provides an entertaining, vivid and popular account of things far-away, strange and exotic. However it is clear that he intends that his status and authority as a medical man should enhance the credibility of his testimony. Before the development of formal anthropology, who better to describe the differences between the varieties of humankind than a trained physician? Skilled in observing the characteristics of European man, he could readily identify how other races departed from this norm. Savage's book should therefore be seen as contributing to the development of the genre of physician-anthropology, which with the works of authors such as Prichard, Lawrence and Wells was to enjoy a considerable vogue in the first few decades of the nineteenth century.[28] As we shall see, Arthur Thomson was to be a distinguished New Zealand example.

Unlike the other doctors this essay is to discuss, Savage seems not to have had any particular political axe to grind when he described the Maoris. Perhaps he wrote to ingratiate himself with Earl Fitzwilliam, to whom the book is dedicated and in whose hands Savage's career in the public service lay. The amusement of Fitzwilliam certainly seems to have been a principal motive for Savage taking a young Maori man with him back to England. If this was indeed his intention, he seems to have succeeded since all the charges against him were set aside and he was given a position with the East India Company.[29] For our purposes Savage's image of the Maoris as Noble Savages (or as near as makes little difference) provides an illustration of how the eighteenth-century's conventional perceptions of the Maori survived into the nineteenth. We shall see other examples later in this essay. Savage's very appreciative assessment of the indigenous people of New Zealand is also useful as a benchmark with which to assess the medical views of the Maori to be found later on in the century. All will be found to be less positive than Savage's, each differing from his in its own distinctive way.

Missionary medicine: Romantic savages

In 1834 the warship *Alligator* was sent to New Zealand from New South Wales on a punitive expedition against a Taranaki Maori tribe who had killed some of the crew of a whaling ship and taken some more prisoner.[30] In a skirmish between the tribesmen and an assault force sent from the *Alligator*, a local chief was wounded. He was treated for his injuries by the ship's surgeon, William Marshall.

Marshall reported himself very impressed by the chief's dignity and bravery and by the rapid recovery he made. Wounds, Marshall wrote, the like of which would have 'killed outright any man with a European constitition' seemed to cause the chief, 'little inconvenience beyond the weakness incidental to excessive haemorrhage'.[31] Such resilience was, according to Marshall, typical of the Maoris. He attributes their remarkable powers of recuperation to the fact that their bodies were not weakened by the European luxuries of liquor and too much food:

> They whose diet consists chiefly of fruit and vegetables, whose drink is that of creation's own providing, in its simplest and purest form, water from the river or brook, and that drank only seldom and in small quantities, may well be expected to have constitutions that can stand up against almost any violence.[32]

Moreover the Maoris are spared 'unwholesome occupations and sedentary pursuits'. They suffer from neither the vices nor the anxieties of civilisation. They are closer to nature and accordingly one finds in their bodies the *vis medicatrix naturae* raised to its greatest possible perfection.

In some ways Marshall's account is very similar to John Savage's. However it is important to note that, despite these similarities, Marshall's view of the Maori differs in several crucial respects fom the ideal of the Noble Savage. The view that the South Pacific islanders were, in their natural state, among the most fortunate of mankind did not greatly appeal to those who saw it as the Europeans' duty to improve the lot of primitive peoples by introducing them to Christianity.[33] Nor, although they placed great emphasis on the depravity of pagan peoples, were the missionaries altogether happy with the opposite idea of the Ignoble Savage. Utter ignobility could not be conceded without weakening the missionaries' case since it might carry the unfortunate implication that primitive peoples were incapable of responding to civilising influences or to the uplifting message of Christianity.[34] Apologists for Church activity in the South Seas often preferred the modified version of noble savagery that Bernard Smith has termed the idea of the 'Romantic Savage'.[35] Certainly the Polynesians were unhappy and benighted pagans but pagans with real, actual and potential, positive qualities – qualities which could be redeemed and complimented by Christianity and by civilisation. Mary Mitford expressed the ideal very vividly in her poem *Christina* which is set on Pitcairn island, and which was published in 1811.[36] She saw arising in the South Seas a new social order founded upon a judicious blend of the benefits of Christian civilisation wih the sturdy virtues of the natural savage life.

Marshall is a vigorous apologist for the work of the missionaries in civilising and converting the Maori. He provides what is virtually a medically evidenced and authorised version of the notion of the Maoris as Romantic Savages. As well as appreciating the vigour of their constitutions, he admires the tall, athletic physique of the Maori warriors. He comments favourably on their individual heroism and bravery under fire and notes how, when abandoning a besieged village, they, in unconscious imitation of the best traditions of the British Navy, evacuated women and children first. He finds their dress elegant and their houses beautifully and skilfully made. Moreover they are not devoid of a moral sense for they have a childlike faith in fair play and personal integrity. Even their superstitions are not wholly depraved, indicating that the Maori have the potential for a higher spirituality. They merely lack enlightenment:

> Amid the thick mist of native superstitions, glimmerings of light, though dim, and faint, and transient, are here and there visible: and among other truths, the difference between soul and body seems to have been discerned among the people, before the preachers of the Gospel had instructed them – and the separate existence of the soul after death appears to have been generally acknowledged.[37]

To be sure Marshall regards the Maori as depraved and addicted to vice. This is the most significant difference between his view and Savage's. They are 'unhappy barbarians' in the 'forlorn condition of savages'.[38] They are ignorant and greedy, sometimes to the point of heartlessness. Ill treatment of slaves and women is commonplace. Warfare is endemic between the tribes. The missionaries work 'amid scenes of blood' and 'surrounded by the habitations of cruelty'.[39] But Marshall continuously emphasises that, with proper moral and spiritual guidance, the Maori is capable of much better things. He angrily rebuts the notion that they are 'irreclaimable'.[40]

A recurring motif of Marshall's text is the argument that the depravity of the Maori is actually less than that of the worst sort of European whom 'civilisation separated from Christianity hath rendered a hundred thousand times more savage than the most degraded of the aboriginies of heathen land'.[41] He is bitterly critical of the brutal and ill-disciplined military action taken by the *Alligator* against the Cape Egmont *hapu*.[42] On that occasion 'how superior was the conduct of the New Zealand savages' to that of the British, so-called Christians.[43]

Marshall is convinced that European contact has been far from an unmixed blessing to the Maoris. The prostitution trade with European ships has caused, he argues, much infertility and ill-health among the Maori women. Secular commerce in general has exercised a baneful influence over the New Zealanders: 'Beyond thinning the forest of its stately inhabitants and propagating among the natives a filthy and terrible disease, commerce, while returning enriched herself from the ports of New Zealand, left the country unimproved by her visitations, and its aboriginal tenantry, not a little injured.'[44]

Marshall explicitly acknowledges that the purpose of his publishing an account of his observations in New Zealand is to provide support, financial and political, for missionary activity. The profits from his book are to go to the Church Missionary Society 'for the immediate extension of their work in New Zealand'.[45] The book's preface is addressed to Lord Glenelg, Secretary of State for the Colonies. His Lordship is entreated to use his political influence 'on behalf of the natives of New Zealand, and the Aborigines of barbarous countries generally . . . who have hitherto experienced neither justice nor mercy at our hands as a nation'.[46]

The timing of Marshall's publication is very significant. In 1836 the Church Missionary Society was deeply involved in a full-scale dispute with the New Zealand Association who had newly published plans for the establishment of large British settlements in New Zealand.[47] Both sides assailed the Colonial Office with a constant bombardment of pamphlets and deputations. The New Zealand Association argued that, apart from promoting the general good of imperial expansion, secular European settlement would be beneficial to the Maori since it would display to them the advantages of civilisation. The Church Missionary Society argued that increased intercourse with Europeans would be bad for the Maori, as it had been bad for the American Indian and the Australian Aborigine. A large influx of settlers would dilute the beneficial effects of missionary activity and would weaken the civilising influence which the missionaries currently exercised. Large-scale emigration to New Zealand should not be allowed. Marshall's text is explicitly a part of this sustained effort by the Church Missionary Society to persuade Parliament and the Secretary of State to block the New Zealand Association's plans. Indeed Marshall has to apologise for 'following so vast a train into the presence and chamber of the King's minister, with humble petition to add to theirs'.[48]

The medical evidence Marshall provides supports the missionary cause in two ways. Firstly it demonstrates that the Maoris are not essentially or irredeemably degenerate and so the attempt to Christianise them is not futile. Secondly it illustrates that contact with secular Europeans has already been actually disadvantageous for the Maori. This is an important political point since the Church Missions were frequently criticised, both in New Zealand and elsewhere, for needlessly and selfishly impeding the development of trade and secular European settlement.[49] Marshall argues that when the missionaries oppose settlement they are motivated by what is best for the Maori. The influence and power of the missions ought to be increased so that the Maori may be better protected from the wrong sort of European and from unscrupulous exploitation.

Marshall identifies two principal instruments of British expansionism as deleterious to the welfare of native peoples and therefore less deserving of the Secretary of State's support than missionary activity. The first is imperial military might, which the futility of the Cape Egmont intervention indicts: 'The two parts of [my] narrative will be found to exhibit, in remarkable contrast, the very opposite effects produced, by a Christian mission, upon the minds and morals of the natives; and upon their welfare and propriety, by a military expedition.'[50]

It was politically astute of Marshall to argue that missionaries pacified better than soldiers since the Colonial Office was deeply concerned that providing military protection for a new British colony in far-away New Zealand would be expensive.[51]

Marshall's other target was political economy. The fashionable theories of Adam Smith and Ricardo, as modified into a theory of systematic colonisation by Edward Wakefield, provided much of the rationale employed by the New Zealand Association in support of their settlement plans.[52] To Marshall such notions are merely ungodly weapons in the battle between Mammon and the Church for the souls of the Maori:

> As poison in the prescription of a wise physician is calculated to contribute to the recovery of the patient, so the blight that has withered the speculations of political economists, as to the best way of raising the tribes of the heathen from their moral and social degeneration, into the ranks of civilised beings, and to a place among the nations of the earth, may serve to exhibit in a more perfect contrast, how superior is the foolishness of God to the wisdom of man.[53]

One should bear in mind that, in terms of the history of New Zealand, 1834 – when Marshall made his observations – is very early indeed.[54] New Zealand was the last of the dominions to be annexed and settled. Before the missionaries arrived in 1815, the entire European settlement consisted of a few traders who supplied European goods to the Maori and shipped timber, flax and some Maori agricultural produce to New South Wales. They also provided food, rum and Maori women for the crews of visiting whaling ships. The European population probably did not go above two thousand until Britain officially claimed sovereignty in 1840.

By the 1830s and 1840s it was widely accepted, both in Britain and abroad, that contact with the civilised nations generally had seriously harmful effects on indigenous races.[55] The population numbers of native peoples were acknowledged to decline, even to the point of extinction, on their being brought under European domination. The reasons for this were a matter for considerable debate. However many observers were prepared to attribute at least some of this decline directly to the active hostile agency of the Europeans. Public disquiet at the barbaric treatment meted out to the aboriginal population in Australia led to a report by a Select Committee of the House of Commons in 1837.[56] The Colonial Office was severely censured for allowing, as the report put it, 'the Tasmanians to be shot like dogs'. Furthermore, with the setting-up of the Aborigines Protection Society in 1837, there was now a vocal and organised philanthropic lobby in London which had as one of its main concerns the welfare of the indigenous peoples of the Empire.[57] It was politically expedient for the British Government to at least appear to try harder in its newest colony, New Zealand. Thus, although the New Zealand Company (as it later became) was eventually allowed to continue with its settlement plans, the missionaries' attempt to Christianise and protect the Maori received, as Marshall had hoped, much early support from the imperial authorities. The Colonial Office also tried to use its own political resources to prevent the European traders and settlers from indulging in the worst excesses of exploitation, appropriation and brutality. Early governors were charged to protect the interests of the Maori as one of their principal priorities.[58]

From the very beginnings of the mission activity in New Zealand, the missionaries provided some degree of backwoods or domestic medical care for Maoris as an incentive for them to attend the missions. However the first medical missionary, so-called, did not arrive until 1837, when Dr Samuel Ford set up a medical mission near what is now Auckland.[59] In 1842 Lady Martin opened the first hospital for Maoris at Judges Bay in the North Island.[60] Apart from regarding the hospitals as instruments of Christian charity, the missionaries also hoped that they would facilitate conversion. Maoris could be exposed to sustained divine ministry during prolonged periods of sickness and convalescence when, it was hoped, they would be particularly susceptible.[61]

The early missionary doctors accepted the fact that the Maoris were declining in numbers. They attributed this decline to the effects of their persistence in sin and paganism. They pointed to promiscuity, the practice of infanticide, and the continuation of warfare between the tribes as the principal causes of the Maoris' imminent downfall as a people. However the missionaries also attributed some blame to those Europeans who did not acknowledge the rightful hegemony of the missionaries and traded with the Maoris in alcohol and guns or otherwise exerted a baneful moral influence over them. The answer, according to the medical missionaries, lay in more missionary activity, limiting immigration and stricter theocratic control over the European community.[62]

Imperial medicine: amalgamating savages

As the size of the European population increased, from 1840 onwards, the imperial government adopted a policy of what was termed 'racial amalgamation'.[63] By selectively incorporating the Maori into European institutions, giving them certain legal and civil rights, and re-educating them in European ways, it was hoped both to subdue the tribes to the European hegemony and to prevent their total degradation in the manner of the Australian Aborigines. Amalgamation was a policy designed to achieve imperial ends peacefully, placating the philanthropic lobby in London and avoiding the expense of sending large numbers of imperial troops to New Zealand.

Medical institutions and medical knowledge both functioned as tools of this policy. As one of his first acts as Governor, Sir George Grey, appointed in 1846, requested authority from the Colonial Office in London to use imperial funds to set up hospitals in New Zealand.[64] These were to be open to both Maori and European patients.[65] This policy of a fully integrated hospital provision is, as far as the present author is aware, unique in British colonial administration, and illustrates the determination of the Colonial Office to pursue the amalgamation policy. However it also illustrates how selective this policy was since it was considered desirable to incorporate the Maori into hospitals as patients while simultaneously refusing them access to those institutions which held genuine political power in the colony. In other words, paradoxically the hospitals played a key role in Grey's amalgamation policy precisely because they were perceived as institutions which were marginal to the overall administrative apparatus of the colonial state.[66]

Grey's requests were granted and colonial hospitals were established in Auckland, Wellington, Wanganui and New Plymouth. The Wellington Hospital opened in 1847 and admitted forty-five in-patients in its first half-year, twenty-nine of whom were Maori. One of the acknowledged purposes of the hospital was to educate the Maori in European ways. In the original admission book it is recorded with evident pride that an early patient refused 'to go out in the blankets in which he was admitted and has bought himself a new suit'.[67] Just as the missionaries hoped that their hospitals would inculcate Christianity, Grey hoped that his would encourage civilisation.

In March 1848, Grey wrote again to the Colonial Secretary in London:

> In my previous despatches to your Lordship upon the subject of the efforts which are being made at once to gain the attachment and to promote the civilisation of the Natives, I stated my belief that very good effects would spring from the establishment of these hospitals and I think that your Lordship will find from the enclosed interesting report that the anticipations I formed are likely to be fully realised.[68]

The report was from Dr John Fitzgerald, Superintendent of the Colonial Hospital at Wellington. Fitzgerald wholeheartedly confirmed that the plan of treating both races together in the same wards had had admirable results. 'Since the hospital opened,' he wrote, 'nothing but harmony has existed between both races.'[69] Fitzgerald recorded that Maoris came from far and wide to the hospital. He suggested that a hospital visiting committee be set up with a large Maori representation upon it. The hospitals were held to display, in a microcosm, the results being achieved throughout New Zealand with the policy of racial amalgamation.

To mark the imperial government's appreciation of the work carried out by the hospital and the co-operation given by the Maoris, the Colonial Secretary presented to the hospital a collection of books and a large engraving of Queen Victoria. To celebrate the reception of the gifts, Dr Fitzgerald arranged an entertainment in the hospital for the local Maori chiefs. The engraving was hung at the end of the room 'to impress the natives with some idea of the pomp and circumstance attendant on Her Majesty'.[70]

As we know from Professor Ranger's work on Southern Africa, doctors were often seen by the nineteenth-century colonial authorities as a vital part of their apparatus of authority and control.[71] Western medicine was a key weapon in the campaign to weaken indigenous culture and promote allegiance to European institutions and modes of thought. When Grey moved to South Africa in 1854, Fitzgerald went with him. Grey sent him to the frontier to practise what was termed 'disinterested medicine' and to wean the natives from witchcraft.[72] In fact, Fitzgerald was not at all disinterested. He was, for example, expected to supply Grey with military intelligence. In New Zealand Fitzgerald's testimony was used by Grey to congratulate the Colonial Office upon the correctness of their policy of racial amalgamation and to convince them of the success of Grey's implementation of it in New Zealand.

Another important figure in New Zealand medicine at this time was Arthur S. Thomson, who gained his M.D. from Edinburgh in 1833.[73] In August 1847, he came to New Zealand as the Surgeon-Major to the 58th regiment of Foot. He remained in the colony for eleven years. In 1854 he published a detailed description of the Maori and their diseases.[74] His treatise still retains some touches of noble or romantic savagery. He writes, for example, that 'clothed in native dress the New Zealander looks like a lion of the forest; in European clothes he is squat and vulgar'.[75] However, unlike Marshall, he does not admire the Maoris' dwelling-places. Indeed he regards their huts as being worse than dog kennels.

The medical evidence Thomson presents is conspicuously pertinent to a favourable assessment of the success of the policy of racial amalgamation. He is evidently concerned to demonstrate that the Maoris have benefited from European contact. A good exemplification of this is to be found in his description of the disease *lepra gangraenosa*,, a form of leprosy, which he holds to be new to medical science and peculiar to the Maori.[76] Thomson believes the causes of the disease to be lack of personal cleanliness and indolence of mind and body. No European or half-caste ever suffers from the disease because the mental activity of civilisation is a perfect prophylactic against it. Likewise Maori women living with European men are completely immune. And thanks to the civilising European influence, the disease is in decline even among Maoris:

> It is a pleasing task for me to record that commerce has introduced considerable activity of mind and body among the New Zealanders living near the English settlements, and among those who can reach them in canoes and small vessels . . . What has been the consequence? The disease I have now endeavoured to describe is becoming rare; probably in twenty years more, civilisation and her handmaidens, industry and cleanliness,

> will have extended themselves to the tribes in the interior of the country, and . . . the Lepra Gangaenosa may become extinct.[77]

Thomson is very concerned to refute the accusation, made, as we have seen, by Marshall among many others, that some of the apparent infertility among Maori women was the result of venereal infections introduced by Europeans. He maintains that gonorrhoea occurred in New Zealand before western contact, and in any case, he claims, venereal disease is very rare in the European community, even among the soldiers. Furthermore the Maori suffer only mildly from syphilis. He remarks that neither he nor any of his medical colleagues has seen a native severely disfigured as a result of venereal infection. He categorically denies the claim, made by Marshall, that the Maori prostitutes die young. Rather, he asserts, they disappear back to their villages in the interior where they are much sought after as wives because it is evident to their menfolk that even in the degraded position of a prostitute they have acquired some superior civilised habits by living among Europeans.[78]

The substance of Thomson's report is a vindication of European involvement in New Zealand, and of imperial native policy, which he maintains has been 'from the first . . . just, generous, and benevolent'.[79] He states explicitly that one of the objects of his memoir is 'to place on record, before years have placed proof out of the question, that the decay of the New Zealanders is not the work of the early settlers':

> Good men in England have attributed the frequent extinction of certain aboriginal races to the cruel conduct, and the unchristian treatment of the early settlers among them. The hands of the white men in America, Van Dieman's Land, New Holland, and Algeria, may not be clean from this imputation; but not so the pioneers of European colonisation in New Zealand.[80]

Rather he argues that their decline is due to the Maoris themselves for they have persistently violated 'those natural laws that God has made for the propagation and increase of the human species'.[81] They are guilty of promiscuous sexual intercourse, of infanticide, of intermarrying with close relatives, especially, he says, scrofulous ones, of neglecting the sick in general and the proper usage of medicine in particular.

Governor Grey included a version of Thomson's report in one of his despatches to London and it was eventually printed in the Parliamentary Papers on New Zealand. It was much quoted in assessments of the effectivenesss of imperial policy towards the Maori even into the twentieth century.[82] We can see from the history of Thomson's report, as we saw from the history of Fitzgerald's, that the testimony of doctors had a crucial significance in imperial debate and polemic. Because of the central importance of questions of native welfare to claims as to the overall success of imperial policy in the mid-and-late nineteenth century, favourable medical testimony was particularly valuable to the imperial administrators as they sought to defend and legitimate their activities against the scrutiny of the strong philanthropic lobby in London. Thomson is well aware of the significance of the evidence he gives. The correct elucidation of the reasons for the decline of the Maori is, he was later to write, a matter of 'the honour of England'.[83]

In a book published on his return to England, Thomson provided an even more explicit and detailed medical defence of the policy of racial amalgamation. It should of course be always borne in mind that the policy of amalgamation, although it purported to treat the Maori as, at least potentially, the equal of the settler in questions of civil rights, was in fact firmly based upon the assumption of the absolute superiority of the European and his institutions. Thomson provides biological legitimation for this assumption: 'It was ascertained, by weighing the quantity of millet seed skulls contained and by measurements with tapes and compasses, that the New Zealand heads are smaller than the heads of Englishmen. Consequently the New Zealanders are inferior to the English in mental capacity.'[84] Thomson does however believe that the intelligence of the Maori will be improved by the stimulations of commerce. Already he claims Maori heads are getting bigger.

Thomson explicitly refutes the notion, so central to Marshall's view of the Maori, that the human race degenerates physically under the conditions of civilisation. He produces the results of experiments he has carried out on the relative strengths of the Maoris and the Europeans. It is the Maori that is shown to be the weaker:

> Persons who delight in thinking that the human race degenerates physically after years of civilisation, will be surprised to hear that the New Zealanders are not equal to the English in bodily strength. The extent of this inferiority may be put down at fifty pounds; for in a trial of strength, New Zealand men raised on average 367 pounds an inch from the ground, and Englishmen 422 pounds.[85]

Thomson presents racial amalgamation as a law of nature and a beneficial one:

> In all conquests, whether by the mind or by the sword, which have terminated in good to the weaker party, the conquerors have invariably amalgamated with the conquered; and this is most necessary among the New

> Zealanders, as their rapid decrease is much aggravated by their breeding in . . . It is therefore satisfactory to find that Caucasian blood already flows in the veins of two thousand of the native population . . . The New Zealanders are melting away; but they are not lost, they are merging into another and a better class.[86]

He describes the half-castes as a 'noble and beautiful race' requiring only education to develop the force and power of their minds. They have something of the vigour of hybrids. For example, they are, Thomson asserts, singularly free from scrofula, which he has earlier termed the 'diseased taint of Maori blood'. The product of the New Zealand melting pot will not however be 'coffee coloured people by the score':

> With regard to physical appearance, the law of amalgamation is that the type of the less numerous shall be lost in that of the greater number . . . As the Anglo-Saxon settlers in New Zealand must soon outnumber the aborgines, the features of the Maori race will disappear from among the half-caste, although traces of their blood will occasionally be seen in families after many generations.[87]

In other words Thomson provides medical authority for the conclusion that the imperial policy of educating the Maori, giving them certain civil rights, if not quite full citizenship, and at the same time, gradually buying up their land and encouraging European settlement, will guarantee a smooth transition to an all-white New Zealand and will lead to a peaceful end to the Maori problem.

The doctor had an almost unique claim to privileged, disinterested expertise on racial questions, partly through his status as a man of science and partly because of the close contact he legitimately maintained with the indigenes. Thomson, for example, has to acknowledge that his description of the character of the Maori is less favourable than that usually given. He is however able to buttress the credibility of his account by claiming that it has been drawn up from personal observation among them 'in their days of happinesss and sorrow, and in their hours of sickness and death'.[88] Medical testimony has, therefore, the authority both of objective science and intimate personal experience.

Thomson's book is a comprehensive, authoritative and very detailed account of New Zealand, its indigenous inhabitants and its European settlements. It is, as mentioned earlier, an important contribution to the nineteenth-century genre of physician-anthropology. It remains to the present day a useful anthropological document.[89] There can be no doubt about Thomson's assiduity as an original investigator and as a collator of the best available information. In sum, his observation of the Maori was as scientific as that of any contemporary observer of non-European peoples. There can, however, equally be no doubt that, in several instances, this authoritative and scientific text serves the interests of imperial policy and legitimation.

It should be noted that it was not only imperial native policy to which Thomson's medical evidence was particularly and conspicuously relevant. The expertise of the doctor had a key significance in supporting several aspects of imperial expansionism. For example, both the Governor and the immigration companies wished to attract more settlers in order more firmly to establish European domination and to increase military security. Here again the evidence of doctors was crucial. A clean bill of health was essential in establishing the attractiveness of the colony. As an appendix to a chapter explicitly addressed to prospective immigrants, Thomson provides climatic and statistical evidence to show that New Zealand is healthier than both England and the other possible settler destinations such as Australia, Canada or the USA.[90] It was thus a good investment, medically speaking, to spend the extra time and money required to make the longer journey to New Zealand.

Settler medicine: dying savages

The 'humanitarian' or 'Philo-Maori' policy of the Colonial Office was not the only native policy in mid-nineteenth-century New Zealand. From the late 1840s on, the Maori question was inceasingly a cause of tension between the settlers and the colonial authorities.[91] Both the colonial authorities and the settlers wanted to impose European hegemony over the Maori. Many of the settlers' leaders were however impatient at the gradualist pace of imperial policy – a policy which, in any case, they saw as unduly sympathetic and concessionary to Maori customs and institutions. They wished to pursue hegemony more vigorously – to impose English law more directly.

As interracial relations worsened in the 1850s and 1860s, the settlers' leaders became more outspokenly hostile to the Maori people and their indigenous culture. To many settlers the idea that the Maori were on the way to extinction was not an altogether unwelcome one.[92] Their preferred image of the Maori became what Howe has termed the idea of the 'Dying Savage'.[93] The imperial authorities and the missionaries continued to urge that the best object was to educate and civilise the Maori so that one day they, or their mixed-race descendants, might be able to take up a place in white society. Some settlers, however, argued that if they were dying out then there was no point in spending time and money on such a task. The Maori would all be gone before they were properly equipped for the exercise of civil responsibility. This was stated quite explicitly by a settler committee which met in Auckland in 1851.[94] Their principal demand was that absolute control of all the internal affairs of the colony should be transferred to the settler community without any interference whatsoever from the imperial government. In particular they wanted complete control over native affairs. Then there would be no more nonsense about educating them to become constitutional equals. The committee pointed to the Maoris'

> total ignorance on almost every subject of knowledge which qualifies for the exercise of political rights – their want of acquaintance with the nature and principles of the British Constitution . . . Nor can your committee conceal from themselves the fact that, owing to causes over which they have no control, the native race is fast becoming extinct, and that there is no prospect of their becoming as a body sufficiently enlightened for the exercise of political privilege before the time of their extinction shall arrive.[95]

One of the roots of the interracial tension was land.[96] The Treaty of Waitangi had recognised the Maoris' title to their tribal lands and in the 1850s they still owned large areas, especially in the interior of the North Island. Colonial Office policy was to try to encourage the chiefs to sell in an orderly gradual way. However sections of the settler community wanted land more quickly. The Wellington Committee saw supremacy over the Maori as the key to releasing land for further settlement. They resolved that: 'The waste land of the colony ought to be placed at the disposal of the colonists, to be administered in such a manner as the Legislature may from time to time see fit.'[97]

Furthermore the settlers were no longer sanguine about the biological prerequisite of the policy of racial amalgamation – miscegenation. As happened in many parts of the Empire the first wave of Europeans was predominantly male and intermarriage took place quite freely with the indigenous population. However once the settler ships of the New Zealand Company arrived, the proportion of women in the European community greatly increased. Furthermore the white community became more complete and self-sufficient and was able to erect social barriers against outsiders. Native wives were not freely accepted into white society.[98] There were, of course, good Victorian reasons for this. A correspondent to an Auckland newspaper challenged the very principle of racial amalgamation in the following fashion:

> Does it mean that we should give our daughters to their sons and take wives of their daughters for our sons? If so what is there to prevent it, except that moral purity cannot descend to the level of animal instincts . . . there can be no companionship . . . between the domestic purity of our wives and daughters and the communism of the native *kainga* where the females were never taught that chastity was a virtue . . . there can be no such social amalgamation until the inferior race shall stand upon the same level in regard to morality and knowledge as ourselves.[99]

As noted above, the doctor often held a privileged position as an expert on native affairs. We have seen that Governor Grey was keen, during his first administration, to adduce medical evidence in support of the policy of amalgamation. However medical expertise could be directed in several ways. The imperial authorities' settler opponents could, with equal facility, find evidence to support their own position, especially since, as Wright-St Clair has pointed out, medically trained men enjoyed very considerable prominence with the immigrant community.[100] They were, by the standards of the time and place, highly educated and well-respected men. They were also often very active in the colony's politics. Doctors were leaders of the settler community and they were thus well placed to make authoritative public pronouncements in its support.

The doctors, who spoke for the settler or Pakeha interest in the period from 1850 onwards, frequently argued, even more strongly than Thomson had done, that the Maori were inherently and biologically inferior.[101] They seized on evidence from craniology and phrenology that Maoris' brains were smaller overall and significantly underdeveloped in vital areas.[102] They did not however hold, as Thomson had done, that civilisation could improve the Maoris' mental capacities. The intellectual inferiority, like the racial effeteness, was quite irredeemable. In 1859, Judge F. D. Fenton gathered much medical evidence in the course of writing his report on the state of the indigenous population.[103] He concluded that the real reason for the dwindling numbers was that the Maori constitution was 'fundamentally rotten'.

That the decline of the Maori was quite inevitable became a central tenet of settler legitimation. There was nothing at all that could be done about it, in the way of social policy or preventive medicine. The prospective extinction of the Maori was merely the working out of an inexorable law of nature. In 1856, Dr Isaac Featherston, Superintendent of Wellington but also a practising physician, put the matter succinctly: 'The Maoris are dying out, and nothing can save them. Our plain duty as good, compassionate colonists is to smooth down their dying pillow. Then history will have nothing to reproach us with.'[104]

From 1850 onwards it became popular to claim that Maori numbers had been dwindling even before European contact – such had been their original depravity and effeteness. William Colenso, for example, argued that Tasman had seen many more Maoris than Cook and that, in the period between Cook's voyages and British annexation, numbers had diminished still more. The decline since 1840 had simply continued an already well-established trend.[105]

The period from 1860 to 1868, with war being actively waged against the Maori by imperial troops, saw the New Zealand politicians under particular pressure to explain themselves to the Colonial Office and the Philo-Maori lobby in London.[106] They were continually harried by the Aborigines Protection Society and its supporters. A series of pamphlets were published under the Society's auspices which expressed scepticism as to the justice of the war and the humanity of its conduct, and impugned the motives of the settlers.[107] In 1868 William Fox, who had been both Native Minister and Chief Minister, published a detailed reply to his Philo-Maori critics.[108] The theory of pre-contact decline had a prominent place in his attempt to defend the record of the New Zealand colonial government. The decline of the Maori could not be the settlers' fault since it had begun before they arrived. Fox argued that the Maori were not disappearing because of any harsh treatment they had received at the hands of the settlers, nor because Europeans had corrupted their morals or given them new diseases. On the contrary they were dying *despite* all the sincere and strenuous efforts which the white community had made on their behalf.[109] Indeed decline had occurred in the face of the kindest and most philanthropic policy ever accorded an indigenous people by their imperial masters.

Fox, addressing a British audience, expressed his sorrow as to the tragic decline of the Maori and his keen regret of the necessity to wage war against them. He praised the nobility of the Maori race and expressed his surprise that such a fine people were so incapable of responding to the challenges of civilisation. In the colony, however, others could afford to be less flattering and more complacent. William Travers, lawyer, politician and naturalist, speaking in Wellington in 1869, described the Maori as 'a race of savages, barbarous beyond conception, and practising rites of so foul a kind that the very existence of such rites was often doubted by modern writers'.[110] He continued:

> If, by the intrusion of the vigorous races of Europe, smiling farms and busy marts are to take the place of the rough clearing and hut of the

> savage, and the millions of a populous country, with the arts and letters, the matured policy, and the ennobling impulses of a free people are to replace the few thousands of the scattered tribes now living in an apparently aimless and unprogressive state, even the most sensitive philanthropist may learn to look with resignation, if not with complacency, on the extinction of a people which, in the past had accomplished so imperfectly every object of Man's being.[111]

As one might predict, the changing political climate also affected medical institutions. From the time that responsibility for the hospitals was transferred to the provincial councils, one of their original functions – that of implementing imperial Maori policy – was redundant.[112] Furthermore the settler authorities were always reluctant to spend the colony's money on Maori welfare.[113] As early as 1848, Dillon Bell, who was to become Native Secretary, went to the extent of arguing that it was a waste of money building hospitals for the Maori anyway.[114] The Wellington Hospital fell into disrepair and plans were afoot to close the one in New Plymouth.[115] One of the reasons adduced in support of this abandonment of a Maori health policy was that they were too effete to benefit from medical care. This was always an extreme position, explicitly refuted by many doctors, but it graphically illustrates that in terms of medical perception of the Maori, we have come a long way from Mr Marshall and his Romantic Savages, hardly inconvenienced by apparently mortal wounds.[116]

By the 1880s New Zealand, or at least its larger towns, had all the social trappings of a full-fledged British colony including well-established learned and scientific societies. But the land and hegemony question still rumbled on.[117] The Maoris were not yet quite subdued. The writ of the Wellington government still did not run over the whole of the country. Tension still existed along the boundary between the settlers' land and that of Kingite Maoris. Moreover interracial relations continued to be soured by resentment over the land confiscation which had followed the Waikato war and over the wholesale alienation of Maori land which the Native Lands Court had facilitated.[118]

The Pakeha, now in ascendancy, would brook no sustained opposition. In Taranaki the Maori prophet Te Whiti successfully organised passive resistance against European encroachment. In 1881 John Bryce, the Native Minister, rode on his community at Parahaki with 1,500 armed men. Te Whiti was captured and transported to the South Island where he and his lieutenant were held without trial for two years. The lands his followers had occupied were released for European settlement.[119]

In the eighties therefore the settlers were still actively engaged in forcibly subduing the Maori to the European hegemony. Moreover they were doing so in the face of a newly sophisticated and knowledgeable opposition. The Maoris were much better politically organised and educated than ever before.[120] Moreover they now had skilled Pakeha help in presenting their case both in Wellington and in London. Several Maori leaders petitioned Queen Victoria for protection, restitution and self-government. In the metropolitan capital the Aborigines Protection Society was still very active in publicising the 'Groans of the Maori'.[121] Members of the imperial parliament were occasionally moved to question their colleagues in Wellington as to the justice of their native policy.[122] The continued sensitivity of the colony's politicians to criticism on the Maori question may be gauged from the fact that when in 1883 the Philo-Maori historian G. W. Rusden published a history of New Zealand which contained some adverse criticism of the conduct of the Maori war, John Bryce sued him for libel.[123] One may conclude that New Zealand politicians still felt the need for polemic resources with which to defend and justify themselves.[124]

In Wellington the prestigious Philosophical Society provided a public platform from which the full authority of modern medical science could be brought to bear upon the matter of European dominance and racial relations in New Zealand. In 1882 Alfred Newman, M.B., M.R.C.P., former president of the Society and soon to be a Member of Parliament, took the opportunity to present the most detailed and argued medical justification of the settlers' position.[125] The text of his talk was later reprinted in the *Transactions* of the New Zealand Institute (later to become the Royal Society of New Zealand).[126]

Newman devoted the early part of his lecture to establishing that the Maoris were indeed very rapidly declining in numbers. He agreed with earlier authors that the beginning of the Maoris' decline had not been simultaneous with the arrival of the white man. Their numbers had been falling before any contact with Europeans had been made, due to their native barbarism and inherent degeneracy. The impact of European civilisation had merely accelerated the process. 'The race is 'run out', it is *effete*; seems thoroughly worn out, and its approaching death has been hastened by the struggles with a newer and a fresher race.'[127]

Arthur Thomson had thought, it will be recalled, that contact with Europeans had brought the Maori the health-giving stimulation of physical and mental activity. Newman, on the other hand, argues that the European yoke has been so lightly placed upon them that the

Maoris now suffer the unfortunate consequences of idleness:

> I agree with certain writers in thinking that *indolence* is also a cause of their decrease. Formerly they were forced to work continually for a living, now they lead the laziest of lives; this laziness generates a host of evils. In the United States it has been observed that negro slaves kept at work increased in numbers, whilst freed negroes steadily decreased.[128]

Neither can they cope with the improved diet to which Europeans have introduced them:

> I am of the opinion . . . that the abundance of easily-got food which they now have in regular supply – food too which is *infinitely more nutritious* than anything they had in the olden times before we came to the country – has led to a state of fatness and general plethora which, as in all the lower animals, leads to a lessened fertility, and in others to absolute sterility.[129]

But the real causes of their decline lay not in diet or external circumstances but in their inherent racial inferiority of mind and body. Their 'weakly constitutioned' bodies provide a 'most nutrient soil' for the germs of tuberculosis. Moreover they lack the mental toughness needed adequately to resist illness, even of a minor sort:

> A want of courage . . . does influence the death-rate: namely the readiness with which they 'throw up the sponge' when attacked by disease. Unquestionably many Maoris die of slight ailments because when attacked they do not fight against the disease and strive to resist its ravages but quietly coil their blankets around them, and lie down passively to die. They seem to have no pluck, and their friends look on in a listless do-nothing way, accepting their fate needlessly.[130]

They are congenitally incapable of the forms of behaviour which are required to maintain health. Here Newman seeks to speak with the full authority of his profession:

> The whole evidence of modern medicine shows, beyond a shadow of a doubt, that the two chief causes of phthisis amongst all nations is the intermarriage of phthisical people, and dwelling on low, damp, ill-drained soils: yet these as the very things which the Maoris seem to prefer doing. Amongst ourselves the awful ravages of phthisis may be either entirely checked or greatly abated, by care, by medicine, by nursing, and by change of climate; of all these the Maori knows nothing . . . he never takes care of himself.[131]

Newman systematically underplays the importance of introduced diseases as causes of the Maoris' decline. Tuberculosis, he insists, predated European contact. Many of the killer diseases of Europe such as smallpox, cholera, plague, yellow fever, typhus, and relapsing fever have never been introduced. He acknowledges that typhoid, scarlet fever, measles and whooping cough have been causes of significant mortality and that lues venerea results in sterility among Maori women as it does among a 'particular class of women in London'. But, on the plus side, leprosy has disappeared due to the above-mentioned improvements in diet and the Maori are only slightly affected by syphilis and diphtheria:

> Looking then at the question as a whole, I am inclined to think that important diseases have not been the chief causes leading to the disappearance of the Maori, but that they have only played a part with others.[132]

In any case a vigorous race would be able quickly to repair its losses from a newly introduced disease. But the Maori do not have the reproductive power to respond in this way.

Newman is anxious to demonstrate that the views he expresses are not peculiar to him but rather reflect the experience of many medical men in New Zealand. He has gathered, he claims, information from a large number of his colleagues. Thus Dr Earle 'dilates on the many hundreds of children that die annually from dysentery and tabes mesenterica'. Dr Spencer, who attends a Maori orphanage, had informed him that although Maori children initially respond well to admission, the improvement does not last. At puberty they get weak again. This is an important departure from earlier views. Thomson had asserted that Maori children flourished when cared for in European homes.[133]

Newman denies that Maori-Pakeha half-castes enjoy hybrid vigour. Instead, like his counterparts in the Southern United States, he maintains that the products of racial interbreeding are physiologically inferior to either original stock:

> I believe that . . . lessened chest capacity is to be found in nearly all New Zealand half-castes. It is true that many have handsome figures and broad shoulders, but their chests are usually of the shallow type seen in consumptives of our own race.[134]

All half-castes die young; few reach the age of forty. Their children are feebler still.

These are arguments pregnant with significance for the policy of racial amalgamation. They also mark another crucial difference between Newman's views and Thomson's:

> Early colonists and many theorists believed that the two races might amalgamate; as a matter of fact the two races will never mingle, and any

> infinitesimal influence that the white race may receive until that not far distant time when the Maori dies out, will thereafter be at once imperceptible.[135]

Newman is quite sanguine about this prospect.

> The disappearance of the race is scarcely subject for much regret. They are dying out in a quick, easy, way, and are being supplanted by a superior race.[136]

Clearly it was not the fault of the settlers that the Maori continued to decline despite everything that had been done for them in the way of a humane policy. The Pakeha could afford to be complacent – no blame attached to them. They had done all they could.

It was quite clear to his audience in Wellington that what Newman was really talking about was the allocation of resonsibility. In the discussion which followed his lecture, James Hector M.D., curator of the Wellington Museum and President of the Philosophical Society, agreed with Newman that the Maoris were in decline. He could not, however, accept Newman's postulation of a natural causation:

> He . . . could not agree with the author in attributing the decrease of the Maori to an inherent tendency to decay. We are really to blame, and chiefly from having induced the Natives to abandon their old habits and customs. We have destroyed their social organisations, and not replaced it with ours . . . There appears to be no reason why the race should have decayed if it had been left alone, or only gradually assimilated to our own, and it is no use trying to excuse ourselves by any other natural law but that of might.[137]

Newman, however, enjoyed influential support. When Dr William Buller F.R.S., resumed the presidency of the Philosophical Society in 1884 he took the opportunity of his presidential address to return to the subject of the decline of the indigenous population.[138] Endorsing much of what Newman had said, Buller placed special stress on the key point of the impossibility of amalgamation due to the half-castes' lack of vigour:

> That the race was doomed he had no doubt whatever . . . The aboriginal race must in time give place to a more highly organized . . . one. This seems to be one of the inscrutable laws of Nature. And, if true to our watchword of progress – social, intellectual, and physical – he could scarcely believe that even the most earnest Philo-Maori would deplore the change.[139]

Buller was quite explicit that no blame should be attached to the settlers for the decline of the Maori. He repeated Featherston's assertion that 'history will have nothing to reproach us with'. All that remained for scholars to do was to collect ethnographic materials before it was too late.

Conclusions

This essay has identified four nineteenth-century images of the Maori. They have been characterised as examples of the Noble, the Romantic, the Amalgamating, and the Dying Savage. We have seen that John Savage's image of the Maori as (almost) Noble Savages was an expression of a prevalent contemporary attitude toward the indigenous inhabitants of the Pacific. It was, in a word, conventional. Savage, trained medical man that he was, understood the Maori in terms of the expectations of the culture from which he sprung and of the audience which he addressed. His account of the Maori was the product of an interaction between his first-hand experience and the social and literary conventions within which he chose to work.

The conventionality of Savage's account is apparent in the mythic character of his portrayal of New Zealand. The texts of Marshall, Thomson and Newman display considerably greater scientificity and empirical content. However they too must be seen as conventional in nature. These authors also chose prevalent contemporary conceptions of indigenous peoples, the ideas of the Romantic and the Dying Savage, as vehicles for their descriptions of the Maori.[140]

Moreover, Marshall, Thomson and Newman all stated, more or less explicitly, that they wrote in support of particular interest groups. One can readily see the extent to which a political agenda structured each author's portrayal of the Maori. Marshall, for example, wrote as a missionary apologist. He was unhappy with the idea of the Maori as a Noble Savage for such a conception granted little improvement for the missionary to accomplish. To him the Maori were unhappy barbarians in pressing need of evangelism. However his account of the Maori also emphasised many positive features since their presence implied that the Maori were worth saving and that the efforts of the missions would not be wasted. The encroachment of the missionaries' traditional opponents – trade and secular settlement – was full of actual and potential medical danger to the Maori. Sterility caused by introduced venereal disease was an indication of this.

Thomson wrote to defend the honour of the British Empire. His view of the Maori was less positive than Marshall's. While Marshall held that savages were stronger than Europeans, Thomson believed that the opposite was true. The white man was in every way superior. Contact with European community was good for the Maori, not only morally but also physically and intellectually. The stimulus of trade, far from making them ill, made them healthier and cleverer. Introduced diseases had not caused infertility. If the Maoris were in decline it was because of their persistence in paganism and barbarism. It was, in other words, their own fault and could not be laid at the door of Europeans in general and the British imperial authorities in particular. The half-castes were vigorous and so the imperial policy of racial amalgamation would eventually succeed.

To Savage the Maori needed no redemption. To Marshall and to Thomson the Maori were, in different ways, redeemable. To Newman they were beyond redemption. They were dying out and nothing could save them. He acknowledged that European diseases had affected the Maori adversely but this was not the major reason for their diminished numbers. They were inherently effete, mentally and physically. No blame for their dwindling numbers attached to the Pakeha community since the decline had begun before European settlement commenced. The half-castes were not vigorous so no amalgamation was possible or desirable.

It is true that certain of the differences between these accounts might be explained in terms of changes in the Maori. Thus when noting that Marshall found their huts admirable whereas Thomson did not, one might bear in mind that, as the demand for flax increased, many Maori *hapu* moved from their traditional dwelling-sites and built more makeshift accommodation nearer their flax grounds.[141] Thomson, therefore, might well have been describing a different quality of hut-building from that seen by Marshall. Similarly one might well conjecture that the effects of introduced disease, alcohol and social disruption made some Maori seem less obviously admirable in Newman's time than had been the case in Savage's or Marshall's.[142] However a comprehensive explanation for the differences between the four images cannot be built along these lines. What change in the Maori diminished the vigour of the half-castes so dramatically between 1855 and 1882? Why did gonorrhoea cause sterility among Maori women in 1834, not in 1855, but again in 1882? Why was trade bad for the Maori in 1834, excellent for them in 1856, yet of no effect at all in 1882? There are no wholly satisfactory realistic answers to these and many similar questions. We are left with no alternative but to accept that Marshall's, Thomson's and Newman's accounts, like Savage's, were not uniquely determined by the objective reality of the Maori. On the contrary each author actively selected both the data and cultural resources with which he constructed his image of the Maori. Moreover their accounts differ from Savage's and from one another's at points of especial significance to the pressing polemical and legitimatory requirements of the groups whose political interest they espouse. It is reasonable to conclude that Marshall's, Thomson's and Newman's images of the Maori were devised so as to serve ideological ends.

As argued earlier, the depictions of the Maori produced by these doctors can be interpreted in a manner very similar to that applied by Bernard Smith to visual images of the South Pacific. One might take as an example Smith's account of the work of William Hodge, the artist on Cook's second voyage. Hodge was trained in the neo-Classical school for landscape painting.[143] During the period of his employment by the Admiralty, it was, however, necessary for him to bear in mind the naval preoccupation with strict accuracy in the drawing of the outlines of coasts and landmarks. Moreover while aboard the *Resolution*, Hodge was in the company of men who took an acute professional interest in the observation of weather and atmospheric effects.

In his painting *The Cape of Good Hope*, executed aboard the *Resolution*, Hodge gives what Smith describes as a 'faithful and naturalistic account of the typical weather conditions prevailing during the expedition's stay at the Cape'.[144] Although the picture contains much fine observation, Smith notes that Hodge did not record exactly what he saw at any single instance. Rather the painting embodies a construct of what 'typical' atmospheric conditions around the Cape were during the period of the *Resolution*'s passage. This construct is obviously a selective one since particular prominence is given in the painting to atmospheric effects of especial interest to his naval companions. The topography of the Cape is depicted accurately but the particular view used in the picture was evidently chosen for its dramatic potential. Various details of the composition are disposed in deference to the conventions of neo-Classical landscape painting.

The Cape of Good Hope may be acknowledged to be the product of a process of careful naturalistic observation. Yet if he had been in the company of geologists rather than navigators, or employed by, say, the Linnean Society rather then the Admiralty, Hodge would have painted another picture, incorporating another set of observations.[145] Hodge's final image is structured by his training as a neo-Classicist, the contemporary taste for the dramatic in landscape painting, and his need to satisfy his employers' interest in accurate topographical drawing and meteorological observation. In other words the painting is the product of an interaction betwen the external world and Hodge's skills and professional commitments.[146] It is constructed so as to serve Hodge's interests in gaining a reputation as a landscape painter and in pleasing his commander on the *Resolution* and his employers in London.

Likewise we may acknowledge that Marshall's, Thomson's and Newman's views of the Maori are the product of empirical observation of their subject matter. In pointing to the degree to which their images are conventional and ideological, we need not cast doubt upon Thomson's claim to have measured Maori skulls or upon Newman's claim to have gathered evidence from a large number of his medical colleagues. Rather we can regard the process of empirical observation and data-gathering as being a selective one. We may see the creative process of producing a scientific text as being structured by cultural assumptions and preconceptions as to the nature of the Maori and by each author's concern for the needs and interests of particular audiences. Newman was evidently especially interested in medical evidence which indicated that the Maoris were inferior and declining and so gave prominence to such evidence in much the same way as Hodge studied the falling of light on the sea and made that a prominent feature of *The Cape of Good Hope*. Unflattering medical evidence served Newman's interests as depiction of atmospheric effects served Hodge's. Just as Hodge chose to paint a view of the Cape which embodied neo-Classical principles, so Marshall chose to understand the sterility of Maori women in terms unflattering to the European and Newman chose to explain the same phenomena in terms unflattering to the Maori. Medical images of the Maori were cultural constructs, expressing not empirical reality itself but a particular relationship between that reality and a specific observer.[147]

As indicated above, a direct parallel can be made between the social use of medical knowledge and the social use of medical institutions. Just as different political agenda produced a variety of images of the Maori, so there were a variety of political purposes to which the hospital was put. To the missionaries native hospitals were instruments of Christian charity and conversion. To Governor Grey and the Colonial Office they were instruments of racial amalgamation. To many settler politicians, by contrast, native hospitals served no useful purpose at all. Thus medical knowledge and medical institutions were alike instruments of social interest and political policy. Medical knowledge was an intellectual equivalent of the tools, weapons, visual images and social institutions which Europeans adapted and devised to accomplish the variety of tasks that their involvement in imperial expansion imposed upon them.[148]

For many years nineteenth-century New Zealand historians seem to have worked with the impression that medical and scientific men were somehow above the struggle and that therefore their testimony need only have its general period assumptions allowed for before it could be used to provide insight into what actually happened in the period under study.[149] In fact, as the above examples demonstrate, the very opposite is the case. Medical evidence was pregnant with implication for crucial aspects of nineteenth-century colonial policy. Medical men were aware of this and some sought to provide political interest groups with legitimatory resources. Thus, far from medical knowledge being essentially or necessarily neutral, it was often ideological, even quite narrowly partisan.

More recently some New Zealand historians have begun to view nineteenth-century scientific and medical knowledge in a more thoroughly historical light. The fullest and most recent discussion of the role of scientific ideas in nineteenth-century colonial racial opinion is to be found in James Belich's convincingly revisionist study of the Maori Wars.[150] Belich points to scientific knowlege having two roles in Victorian Pakeha-Maori relations. One is as part of the general background of ideas which presupposed the inferiority of non-European peoples. The second role is a more active one. Belich depicts nineteenth-century New Zealand actors mobilising scientific ideas in argument and rhetoric. Moreover he identifies particular arguments with specific groups and specific times and places. Thus Belich notes how, as race relations worsened in the mid-nineteenth century, unflattering images of the Maori, supported by the rhetoric of Social Darwinism, began to become popular.

The present essay strongly endorses Belich's view that scientific knowledge was used actively and selectively in support of particular political positions. However the view of scientific knowledge which this essay advances is more active still. It is argued that nineteenth-century scientific knowledge of New Zealand is best regarded not only as part of a background of ideas, nor only as a body of polemical resources, but as something actively made and deployed by historical actors to serve a variety of cultural purposes.

One of the principal virtues of the present study is that it demonstrates that medical images of the Maori legitimated not one but several strands of nineteenth-century imperialism. The fact that the various images were different from each other in politically significant ways indicates the need to regard such accounts as being actively constructed so as to serve social interests. The contemporary background of ideas, the 'total ideology' as Belich terms it, is too blunt an explanatory device to account for the specific distinctions between the different points of view. Indeed the existence of a total ideology of European hegemony could only explain similarities between the views of historical actors and not their differences. Neither can the content of Savage's, Marshall's, Thomson's or Newman's texts be explained solely in terms of a process of selection from the range of metropolitan scientific resource available to New Zealand actors, important though such borrowing undoubtedly was. It is clear that much colonial originality and creativity went into the making of, for example, Thomson's *The Story of New Zealand*.

Perception of the socially active nature of images of the Maori will, it is hoped, act as an antidote to passive and idealist views of the role of scientific knowledge in nineteenth-century New Zealand. Following Belich, Boyd has recently written that the 'hardening of race relations in New Zealand from about 1850 has been attributed to the influence of Social Darwinism as has the myth that the Maori was a dying race'.[151] This essay suggests that the exact opposite of this interpretation is the correct one. It was the hardening of racial attitudes that created the vogue for Social Darwinism and made the Maori into a Dying Savage. Colonial actors were not the dupes nor entirely the creatures of the metropolitan culture. For better or worse, they must be given the credit for having devised their own forms of knowledge to help them attain their own quite distinctive imperial and colonial ends.[152]

Notes

An earlier version of this chapter was given to the Society for the Social History of Medicine's day meeting 'Medicine and Empire' in April 1986. I am grateful to all who made comments on that occasion, as I am to Andy Pickering for remarks on another draft. Throughout the period of preparation of this paper I have been supported by the Wellcome Trust, to whom I wish to express my gratitude. It is also a great pleasure for me finally to have an opportunity publicly to record my thanks to the University of Canterbury, Christchurch and in particular the departments of Botany, Sociology and Philosophy for the hospitality show to me during my visit there in 1977.

1 See, for example, C. Bolt, *Victorian Attitudes to Race*, London, 1971; J. W. Burrow, *Evolution and Society: A Study in Victorian Social Theory*, Cambridge, 1966; D. A. Lorimer, *Colour, Class and the Victorians*, Leicester, 1978.

2 B. Smith, *European Vision and the South Pacific*, Oxford, 1960. See also I. Donaldson and T. Donaldson (eds.), *Seeing the First Australians*, Sydney, 1985.

3 Smith, *European Vision*, p. 7.

4 *Ibid.*, p. 255.

5 In other words, this essay is an application to the history of imperial medicine of the 'strong programme' of the sociology of knowledge: see D. Bloor, *Knowledge and Social Imagery* and B.Barnes, *Interests and the Growth of Knowledge*, London, 1977; see also M. Nicolson and C. McLaughlin, 'Social constructionism and medical sociology; a reply to Mr. R. Bury', *Sociology of Health and Illness*, IX, 1987, pp. 119-26.

6 For an account of the ideas of the Noble and the Ignoble see Smith, *European Vision*, esp. pp. 22-6 and 102-4. Also E. Dudley and M. E. Novak (eds.), *The Wild Man Within: An Image in Western Thought from the Renaissance to Romanticism*, Pittsburgh,

1972; A. Sinclair, *The Savage: A History of Misunderstanding*, London, 1977; P. J. Weston, 'Some images of the primitive before 1800', *History of European Ideas*, I, 1981, pp. 215-36.

7 See D. W. Orchiston and L. C. Horrocks, 'Contact and conflict: the Rowe massacre in early proto-historic New Zealand', *Historical Studies: Australia and New Zealand*, XVI, 1974, pp. 519-30.

8 For example, A. Earle, *A Narrative of a Nine Months Residence in New Zealand in 1827*, London, 1832. For a summary of early nineteenth-century views of the Maori, see P. Adams, *Fatal Necessity: British Intervention in New Zealand 1830-1847*, Auckland, 1977, and M. P. K. Sorrenson, 'How to civilise savages: some "answers" from nineteenth-century New Zealand', *New Zealand Journal of History*, IX, 1975, pp. 97-110.

9 For biographical details of Savage, see G. H. Scholefield (ed.), *Dictionary of New Zealand Biography*, and A. D. McKinlay (ed.), *Savage's Account of New Zealand*, Wellington, 1939, pp. 3-6.

10 J. Savage, *Some Account of New Zealand*, London, 1807, p. 25.

11 *Ibid.*, p. 26.

12 Compare the opinions of the Polynesians discussed in M. Alexander, *Omai: Noble Savage*, London, 1977, and in Smith, *European Vision*, pp. 22-6.

13 Compare J. Hawkesworth, *An Account of the Voyages Undertaken by Order of his Present Majesty for Making Discoveries in the Southern Hemisphere*, London, 1773; L. A. Bougainville, *Voyage autour du Monde par la Frégate du Roi la Boudeuse*, Paris, 1771. One difference between Savage, on the one hand, and Hawkesworth and Bougainville, on the other, is that Savage is very discreet about the sexual mores of the Polynesians.

14 Savage, *Some Account*, p. 87.

15 *Ibid.*, p. 25.

16 *Ibid.*, p. 51.

17 The phrase 'savage of sensibility' is Smith's, *European Vision*, p. 97. It neatly expresses the deistic notion that being closer to Nature heightened the moral and aesthetic senses.

18 Savage, *Some Account*, p. 45.

19 *Ibid.*, p. 51.

20 Most famously Buffon, see C. J. Glacken, *Traces on the Rhodian Shore*, Berkeley, 1967, pp. 663-8, and Lord Monboddo, see Smith, *European Vision*, pp. 70-3.

21 Savage, *Some Account*, p. 43.

22 For example, J. C. Prichard, *Researches into the Physical History of Man*, London, 1813, p. 283.

23 Savage, *Some Account*, p. 88.

24 The poem, which is not Savage's, provides the epigraph for his book. It is printed on the title page and attributed to 'E. H.'.

25 For example, G. Forster, *A Voyage Around the World*, London, 1771; J. R. Forster, *Observations Made During a Voyage Around the World, on Physical Geography, Natural History, and Ethic Philosophy*, London, 1778. See also J. Courtenay, *A Poetical Epistle (Moral and Philosophical) from an Officer at Otaheite*, London 1774, and the discussion in Smith, *European Vision*, pp. 31-3. The views of the two Forsters are discussed in Glacken, *Traces*, pp. 611-18.

26 Savage, *Some Account*, p. 87.

27 *Ibid.*, p. 90.

28 For an introduction to this literature, see K. D. Wells, 'William Charles Wells and the races of Man', *Isis*, LXIV, 1973, pp. 215-25; and *idem*, 'Sir William Lawrence (1783-1867): a study of pre-Darwinian ideas on heredity and variation', *Journal of the History of Biology*, IV, 1971, pp. 319-61.

29 McKinlay, *Savage's*, p. 4.

30 For an account of the *Alligator's* expedition, see I. Wards, *The Shadow of the Land: A Study of British Policy and Racial Conflict in New Zealand 1832-1852*, Wellington, 1968, pp. 11-12.

31 W. B. Marshall, *A Personal Narrative of Two Visits to New Zealand in Her Majesty's Ship 'Alligator'*, London, 1836, p. 186.
32 *Ibid.*
33 See Smith, *European Vision*, pp. 243-47.
34 Both Smith, *European Vision*, and K. R. Howe, 'The fate of the "Savage" in Pacific historiography', *New Zealand Journal of History*, XI, 1977, pp. 137-54, argue that the idea of the Ignoble Savage was characteristic of missionary attitudes to the Maori. This seems to be the case, at least as far as official evangelical propaganda and published missionary opinion is concerned. The missionaries had to argue that there was something in the Maori which was worth protecting and therefore worth restricting European expansion on behalf of. I can find little irredeemable ignobility in the accounts of, for example, Lady Martin, Samuel Marsden, Henry Williams or Richard Taylor. See Lady Martin, *Our Maoris*, London, 1884; J. R. Elder (ed.) *The Letters and Journals of Samuel Marsden 1765–1838*, Dunedin, 1932; L. M. Rogers, *The Early Journal of Henry Williams, Senior Missionary in New Zealand of the Church Missionary Society*, Christchurch, 1961; R. Taylor, *Te Ika A Maui or New Zealand and its Inhabitants*, London, 1855. Taylor's book gives very high praise to 'those commonly regarded as savages'. Taylor asserts 'they possess mind as well as ourselves, and only want similar advantages to obtain an equal enlargement of it', p. 2. This is not to deny that some missionaries with actual and bitter experience in New Zealand did indeed come to see their charges as irredeemable and therefore ignoble in this sense. See for example, the quotation from Nathanial Turner in J. M. R. Owens, *Prophets in the Wilderness: The Wesleyan Mission to New Zealand 1819-27*, Auckland 1974, p. 81; also *idem*, 'Christianity and the Maoris to 1840', *New Zealand Journal of History*, II, 1968, pp. 18-40, for another example of Maoris being regarded as 'incorrigible and irreclaimable'. Nor is it to deny that the many missionaries shared in the general hardening of Pakeha attitudes toward the Maori in the late fifties and sixties, see Note 100 below.
35 Smith, *European Vision*, pp. 247-53.
36 M. R. Mitford, *Christina, the Maid of the South Seas*, London, 1811. Mitford's poem is extensively discussed in Smith, *European Vision*, pp. 248-9.
37 Marshall, *A Personal Narrative*, p. 11.
38 *Ibid.*, p. viii.
39 *Ibid.*, p. 10.
40 *Ibid.*, p. viii.
41 *Ibid.*
42 A *hapu* is a sub-section of a tribe, generally living in one locality.
43 Marshall, *A Personal Narrative*, p. 196. Marshall was not the only critic of this adventure, see Wards, *The Shadow*, p. 13.
44 Marshall, *A Personal Narrative*, p. 304.
45 *Ibid.*, p. i.
46 *Ibid.*, p. ii.
47 For a detailed discussion of the competition between the Church Missionary Society and the New Zealand Association, see Adams, *Fatal Necessity*.
48 Marshall, *A Personal Narrative*, p. ix.
49 For example, Earle, *A Narrative*. Earle voiced the two most common criticisms of missionary activity, namely that the missionaries tamed the Polynesians, destroying their native vigour, and that they obstructed the legitimate activities of secular Europeans. For a missionary reply to Earle see Anon, *A Review extracted from the Protestant Journal*, London, 1833. For a general defence of the missionary involvement in New Zealand, see R. Fitzroy and C. Darwin, 'A letter containing remarks on the moral state of Tahiti, New Zealand, etc', *South African Christian Recorder*, II, 1836, pp. 221-38. See also J. M. R. Owens 'Missionary medicine and Maori health: the record of the Wesleyan Mission to New Zealand before 1840', *Journal of the Polynesian Society*, LXXI, 1972, pp. 418-36.
50 Marshall, *A Personal Narrative*, p. v.
51 See Wards, *The Shadow*,and A. H. McLintock, *Crown Colony Government in New*

Zealand, Wellington, 1958.

52 See E. G. Wakefield, *The British Colonization of New Zealand: Being an Account of the Principles, Objects and Plans of the New Zealand Association*, London, 1837.

53 Marshall, *A Personal Narrative*, p. 304.

54 For interesting accounts of the early history of European involvement in New Zealand, see H. M. Wright, *New Zealand 1769-1840: Early Years of Western Contact*, Cambridge, Massachusetts, 1967; and J. M. R. Owens, 'New Zealand before annexation' in W. H. Oliver and B. R. Williams (eds.), *The Oxford History of New Zealand*, Oxford, 1981, pp. 28-53. For the general history of the colony, see K. Sinclair, *A History of New Zealand*, rev. edn., London, 1980; also Oliver and Williams (eds.), *Oxford History*.

55 See, for example, 'Aristoboulos', *The Universal Destruction of Aboriginal Peoples by Colonizing Nations*, London, 1847. See also G. D. Rowley, *The Destruction of Aboriginal Society*, London, 1972.

56 Aborigines Protection Society, *Report of the Parliamentary Select Committee on Aboriginal Tribes, Reprinted with Comments by the Aborigine's Protection Society*, London, 1837.

57 For the origins and early history of the Aborigines' Protection Society, see R. Rainger, 'Philanthropy and science in the 1830s: the British and Foreign Aborigines' Protection Society', *Man*, XV, 1980, pp. 702-17. See also K. Sinclair, 'The Aborigines' Protection Society and New Zealand: a study in nineteenth-century opinion', unpublished M.A. thesis, University of Auckland, 1946.

58 See A. D. Ward, *A Show of Justice: Racial Amalgamation in Nineteenth-Century New Zealand*, Auckland, 1973; McLintock, *Crown Colony Government*; and R. Dalziel, 'The politics of settlement', in Oliver and Williams (eds.) *Oxford History* pp. 87-111.

59 L. K. Gluckman, *Medical History of New Zealand prior to 1860*, Auckland, 1976, p. 58.

60 Martin, *Our Maoris*, p. 73.

61 *Ibid.*, pp. 73-8 and Marshall, *A Personal Narrative*, p. 260. See also Adams, *Fatal Necessity*, p. 45.

62 For useful accounts of the missionaries' attitudes to the Maori in this period see Adams, *Fatal Necessity* and Owens, 'Missionary medicine'. See also *idem*, 'Christianity and the Maoris'.

63 The best account of the theory and practice of the policy of racial amalgamation is in Ward, *A Show*, Auckland, 1973. See also Sorrenson, 'How to civilise savages'.

64 D. M. Wilson, *A Hundred Years of Healing: Wellington Hospital 1847-1947*, Wellington, 1948, p. 17.

65 It is clear from descriptions of the Wellington and New Plymouth hospitals, that each of these institutions only had two wards, one for males and one for females, see Wilson, *A Hundred Years*, p. 18, and W. H. Skinner, *Pioneer Medical Men of Taranaki*, New Plymouth, 1933, pp. 115-39. See also D. Scott, *The Story of Auckland Hospital 1847-1977*, Auckland, 1977.

66 It should also be noted that the native hospitals were situated in the European towns, that is to say at some distance from the major centres of Maori population. It is difficult therefore to see them as a central part of an enlightened imperial medical policy, see R. T. Lange, 'The revival of a dying race: a study of Maori health reform, 1900-1918', unpublished M.A. thesis, University of Auckland, 1972, p. 46.

67 Quoted in Wilson, *A Hundred Years*, p. 19.

68 *Ibid.*

69 *Ibid.*

70 *Ibid.*, p. 20.

71 T. Ranger, 'Healing in the history of colonial south/central Africa', *Bulletin, Society for the Social History of Medicine*, 23, 1978, pp. 9-10.

72 *Ibid.*, p. 9.

73 For biographical details of Thomson, see Scholefield, *Dictionary*, and A. H. McLintock (ed.), *An Encyclopaedia of New Zealand*, Wellington, 1966.

74 A. S. Thomson 'On the peculiarities in figure, the disfigurations, and the customs of the New Zealanders; with remarks on their diseases, and on their modes of treatment', *British and Foreign Medico-Chirurgical Review*, XIII, 1854, pp. 489-502; XIV, 1854, pp. 461-70; XV, 1855, pp. 520-9.

75 *Ibid.*, XIII, p. 490.

76 *Ibid.*, XIII, p. 496.

77 *Ibid.*, XIII, p. 502.

78 *Ibid.*, XIV, p. 470.

79 *Ibid.*, XIV, p. 461.

80 *Ibid.*, XIV, p. 461.

81 *Ibid.*, XIV, p. 462.

82 See, for instance, the item on Thomson in Scholefield, *Dictionary*.

83 A. S. Thomson, *The Story of New Zealand: Past and Present, Savage and Civilised*, London, 1859, II, p. 283.

84 Thomson, *The Story*, I, p. 81.

85 *Ibid.*, p. 73.

86 *Ibid.*, II, p. 305.

87 *Ibid.*, p. 306.

88 *Ibid.*, I, p. 86.

89 See, for example, J. M. Davidson, 'The Polynesian foundation', in Oliver and Williams, *Oxford History*, pp. 3-27.

90 Thomson, *The Story*, II, p. 322.

91 See J. O. Miller, *Early Victorian New Zealand: A Study of Racial Tension and Social Attitudes, 1839-82*, Oxford, 1958; and Ward, *A Show*; also B. J. Dalton, *War and Politics in New Zealand, 1855-1870*, Sydney, 1967; and H. Miller, *Race Conflict in New Zealand 1814-1865*, Auckland, 1965.

92 As Rev. James Buller suggested, the 'wish was often father to the thought', Buller, *Forty Years in New Zealand*, London, 1878, p. 164. See also Lange, 'The revival of a dying race', p. 71 *et passim*.

93 Howe, 'The fate of the "Savage"', p. 141.

94 The background to, and activities of, this committee are well described in Miller, *Early Victorian*, pp. 148-60.

95 Quoted in *ibid.*, p. 155.

96 See K. Sinclair, *The Origin of the Maori Wars*, Wellington, 1957; and Dalton, *War and Politics*. Note that this essay does not suggest that land expropriation was the principal or only *causus belli*, see A. Ward, 'The origin of the Anglo-Maori wars; a reconsideration', *New Zealand Journal of History*, I, 1967, pp. 148-70; and J. Belich, *The New Zealand Wars and the Victorian Interpretation of Racial Conflict*, Auckland, 1986, pp. 76-80.

97 Quoted in Miller, *Early Victorian*, p. 156.

98 For a description of New Zealand society in the mid-nineteenth century, see J. Graham, 'Settler society', in Oliver and Williams (eds.), *Oxford History*, pp. 112-38.

99 *The Aucklander*, 22 August 1862, quoted in Ward, *A Show*, p. 154.

100 R. E. Wright-St Clair, 'Medical men in early New Zealand politics', *New Zealand Medical Journal*, LXXXIV, 1955, pp. 581-5.

101 It should be noted that in the sixties and especially during Grey's second administration, the attitudes of both missionaries and imperial administrators hardened against the Maori. Grey had become impatient with the failure of his paternalism to guarantee the allegiance of the chiefs. Many missionaries, frustrated at the Maori's continued eclecticism and independence, were convinced that only a show of the supremacy of British arms would convince the Maori of the necessity to acknowledge their backwardness and barbarity. Thus settler opinion became less distinct from that of the other European groups in the colony. See Ward, 'The origin of the Anglo-Maori wars'. The Maori word 'pakeha' was (and is) used by both races to refer to persons of European descent.

102 See Ward, *A Show*, p. 161.

103 F. D. Fenton, *Observations on the State of the Aboriginal Inhabitants of New*

Zealand, Auckland 1859.

104 Quoted in Miller, *Early Victorian*, p. 104. Featherston's classic attempt at legitimation has been quoted so many times it is in danger of becoming hackneyed. However it has not hitherto been pointed out that the remark gained special significance and authority from having been said by a medical man.

105 W. Colenso, 'On the Maori races of New Zealand', *Transactions of the New Zealand Institute*, I, 1868, pp. 1-75.

106 For an account of the interracial conflict, see Belich, *The New Zealand Wars*.

107 See, for example, Anon, *The New Zealand Government and the Maori Wars of 1863-64*, London, 1864.

108 W. Fox, *The War in New Zealand*, London, 1866.

109 *Ibid.*, pp. 257-60

110 W. T. L. Travers, 'On the changes effected in the natural features of a new country by the introduction of civilised races', *Transactions of the New Zealand Institute*, II, 1869, pp. 299-330.

111 *Ibid.*, p. 313.

112 For the development of New Zealand's colonial constitution, see Dalziel, 'Settler society'.

113 See Ward, *A Show*, p. 274 *et passim*.

114 Quoted in Miller, pp. 106-7.

115 For Wellington, see Wilson, *A Hundred Years*, pp. 21-4. For New Plymouth, see Skinner, *Pioneer Medical Men*, p. 139; and G. Lambert, *Peter Wilson: Colonial Surgeon*, p. 185.

116 For the argument that epidemic disease 'need not necessarily act more unfavourably on Natives', see Cusack, 'Memorandum by Dr Cusack on the epidemic of measles among the natives', *The New Zealand Gazette*, 1868, p. 72. Peter Wilson was of the same opinion, see Lambert, *Peter Wilson*.

117 See M. P. K. Sorrenson, 'Maori and Pakeha', in Oliver and Williams, *Oxford History*, pp. 168-93; also *idem*, 'The Maori King movement 1858–1885' in R. M. Chapman and K. Sinclair (eds.), *Studies of a Small Democracy: Essays in Honour of Willis Airey*, Auckland, 1963.

118 For the activities and effects of the Native Land Court, see Ward, *A Show*, pp. 212-17, and M. P. K. Sorrenson, 'Land purchase methods and their effect on Maori population 1865-1901', *Journal of the Polynesian Society*, LXV, 1956, pp. 183-99.

119 This episode is described in some detail in the partisan account of G. W. Rusden, *Auretanga: Groans of the Maori*, London, 1888. See also Ward, *A Show*, and Sorrenson, 'Maori and Pakeha'; and D. K. Fieldhouse, 'Sir Arthur Gordon and the Parihaka crisis 1880-1882', *Historical Studies: Australia and New Zealand*, X, 1961, pp. 30-49.

120 Ward, *A Show*; Sorrenson, 'Maori and Pakeha'; and A. Parsonson, 'The pursuit of mana', in Oliver and Williams, *Oxford History*, pp. 140-67.

121 See Rusden, *Auretanga*.

122 See, for example, question by Hicks-Beach, 13 July 1882, *Hansard*, CCLXXII, 271; and documents in British Parliamentary Papers, *New Zealand, Correspondence etc., Respecting Native Affairs in New Zealand and the Imprisonment of Certain Maoris*, 1882.

123 The book was G. W. Rusden, *History of New Zealand*, Melbourne, 1883. For the arguments used in the court case, see *idem*, *Tragedies in New Zealand in 1868 and 1881*, London, 1888.

124 Defence of their native policy was important to New Zealand politicians for a number of reasons. From the 1850s New Zealand politicians were using the supposed excellence and humanity of their native policy as an argument in support of their claim for a New Zealand sphere of influence in the south and central Pacific islands, see Ross, *New Zealand Aspirations in the Pacific in the Nineteenth Century*, Oxford, 1964, p. 49 *et passim*.

125 For biographical details of Newman: McLintock, *Encyclopaedia*.

126 A. K. Newman, 'A study of the causes leading to the extinction of the Maori', *Trans-*

actions of the New Zealand Institute, XIV, 1881, pp. 459-77. See also *idem*, 'Anniversary address', *Transactions of the New Zealand Institute*, XII, 1879, pp. 433-8.

127 Newman, 'A study', p. 464, emphasis in original.

128 *Ibid.*, p. 470, emphasis in original.

129 *Ibid.*, p. 474, emphasis in original.

130 *Ibid.*, p. 471. Thomson, by contrast, had asserted that 'among the New Zealanders the desire to live was as strong as among other races of men', 'On the . . . New Zealanders', XV, p. 525.

131 Newman, 'A study', p. 466.

132 *Ibid.*, p. 469.

133 Thomson, *The Story*, I, pp. 216-7.

134 Newman, 'A study' p. 475. For similar opinions from the United States, see J. S. Haller, *Outcasts from Evolution: Scientific Attitudes of Racial Inferiority, 1859-1900*, Urbana, 1971; *idem*, 'The negro and the Southern physician; a study of medical and racial attitudes', *Medical History*, XVI, 1970, pp. 238-53; *idem*, 'The physician versus the negro: medical and anthropological concepts of race in the late nineteenth century', *Bulletin of the History of Medicine*, XLVI, 1970, pp. 154-67.

135 Newman, 'A study', p. 476.

136 *Ibid.*, p. 477.

137 'Wellington Philosophical Society', *New Zealand Times*, 25 January 1882.

138 For biographical details of Buller, see Scholefield, *Dictionary*. Buller's title derived from an honorary doctorate, not a medical qualification.

139 W. Buller, 'Presidential address to the Wellington Philosophical Society', *Transactions of the New Zealand Institute*, XVII, 1884, pp. 443-6.

140 In terms of the general pattern of Victorian notions of non-European peoples, the Amalgamating Savage was a variant upon the idea of the Dying Savage.

141 Gluckman, *Medical History*, pp. 169-70. On the other hand there is evidence that some Maori building improved after European contact, see Davidson, 'The Polynesian foundation'.

142 See Ward, *A Show*, p. 222. Note that I am not here postulating large-scale social collapse in the Maori heartlands.

143 Hodge's career is discussed in Smith, *European Vision*, pp. 39-58.

144 *Ibid.*, p. 43.

145 Smith, *European Vision*, gives several examples of how the naval genre of the coastal profile could be adapted so as to display geological information. He also notes how the precision of botanical illustration influenced topographical painting.

146 For an interesting discussion of visual images from the perspective of the sociology of knowledge, see Barnes, *Interests*, pp. 1-10. See also S. Shapin and S.Schaffer, *Leviathan and the Air-Pump: Hobbes, Boyle and the Experimental Life*, Princeton, 1985, pp. 17-19.

147 For an explication of the methodology which underlies this interpretation, see M. Nicolson and C. McLaughlin, 'Social constructionism'.

148 For similar social and instrumental usages of ideas of nature, see C. Smith-Rosenberg and C. Rosenberg, 'The female animal: medical and biological views of woman', in C. Rosenberg (ed.) *No Other Gods: Science and American Social Thought*, Baltimore, 1976; and S. Shapin, 'The politics of observation: cerebral anatomy and social interests in the Edinburgh phrenology disputes', in R. Wallis (ed.), *On the Margins of Science: the Social Construction of Rejected Knowledge*, Keele, 1979. Also M. Nicolson, 'The metastatic theory of pathogenesis and the professional interests of the eighteenth-century physician', *Medical History*, due early 1988. For a general discussion of this literature, S. Shapin, 'History of science and its sociological reconstructions', *History of Science*, XX, 1982, pp. 157-211. For some other ways in which biological knowledge served imperial purposes, see L. H. Brockway, *Science and Colonial Expansion: the Role of the British Botanical Gardens*, New York, 1979.

149 See, for a recent example, M. Hoare 'Medical men and science', in Anon (ed.), *Some New Zealand Contributions to Science and Medicine*, Auckland, 1976, pp. 4-5; and

Howe, 'Missionary medicine'. This tendency is a major blemish on the otherwise very informative, Lange, 'The revival of a dying race', and is a besetting sin of Gluckman, *Medical History*.

150 Belich, *New Zealand Wars*, pp. 321-30. See also Howe, 'The fate of the "Savage"'.

151 M. Boyd 'Racial attitudes of New Zealand officials in Westen Samoa', *New Zealand Journal of History*, XXI, 1987, pp. 139-55.

152 My argument here relates closely to recent discussions of the relation between the periphery and the centre in imperial and colonial science. Belich, in common with other New Zealand historians, largely operates with what one might call a centrifugal theory of nineteenth-century scientific knowledge. Scientific knowledge comes from the metropolis to be applied to the colonies. See G. Basalla, 'The spread of Western science', *Science*, CLIV, 1967, pp. 611-22. However Roy Macleod and Ian Inkster have offered modifications of Basalla's model. R. Macleod, 'On visiting the "moving metropolis"', *Historical Records of Australian Science*, V, 1982, pp. 1-16; I. Inkster, 'Scientific enterprise and the colonial "model": observations on Australian experience in historical context', *Historical Records of Australian Science*, XV, 1985, pp. 677-704. Both of these authors, in rather different ways, stress the importance of local circumstances and initiatives in determining the character and development of even the most apparently dependent colonial scientific enterprises.

CHAPTER FIVE

Sleeping sickness epidemics and public health in the Belgian Congo

Maryinez Lyons

Colonial powers commonly regarded their medical and public health programmes as a form of compensation for the hardships caused by their colonisation of African peoples.[1] By the early 1940s the Belgians were proud of their colonial medical services in the Congo which they considered to be an outstanding feature of their 'civilising mission'. The history of medical services in the Congo is intimately linked to the special campaign to fight epidemic sleeping sickness early this century. That campaign formed the basis both for a public health programme and for the creation of a medical service, since it was, as in many African colonies, the first real effort made by the Europeans to deal with the health of Africans.

Following the British discovery in 1901 of a major sleeping sickness epidemic in Uganda, King Leopold of Belgium invited the recently established Liverpool School of Tropical Medicine to examine his Congo Free State. Alarmed at the high mortality rate in neighbouring Uganda, Leopold feared a demographic collapse in the Congo Free State which would frustrate its economic exploitation. By 1902, the year of his invitation to the Liverpool School, the violent practices of Congo Free State agents had aroused international indignation and condemnation. Leopold was much concerned about his tarnished image and he realised that prompt response to a possible epidemic of sleeping sickness in the territory might help to improve his reputation. From the outset, medical provision for the Congolese was related to economic and political considerations. While the Belgian government, which subsequently took over the running of the Congo from Leopold, tried to avoid further administrative mismanagement, medical provision remained closely related to economic and political objectives.

Declaring the disease to be epidemic in some regions of the State, the Liverpool researchers advised Leopold to take urgent measures to protect areas which they considered to be as yet uninfected – such as the vast northeast, later known as Province Orientale. The 'medicalisation' of the Congolese began soon after this with the sleeping sickness campaign, through which the population was systematically introduced to the idea that European doctors and their medications were the solution to problems of ill health. The Belgian campaign was elaborated and refined over time until by the 1930s it formed the core of the colonial public health programme. However, as one specialist has noted, 'The various colonial sleeping sickness campaigns became a kind of conditioned reflex . . . routine, even a fixation of ideas with the result that all epidemics were fought in stereotyped manner without asking if methods were best from region to region.'[3]

La lutte: the campaign against sleeping sickness

The sleeping sickness campaign operated on two fronts which the Belgians referred to as the *médicamenteuse* and the *biologique*. The former included all the more purely medical aspects such as development and training of staff, European and African; the creation of the annual, itinerant medical missions which by 1930 were examining nearly three million people; the gradual evolution of a network of hospitals and rural clinics, especially in Province Orientale; and research into the disease and possible cures. The second front, *biologique*, was primarily administrative and involved public health measures intended to control the incidence and spread of the disease. The measures within this front were often early attempts at 'social engineering' through the reorganisation, restructuring and control of African societies. Features of this front were the identification and mapping of infected and non-infected zones and the creation of a *cordon sanitaire* to protect mainly non-infected regions such as large portions of the northeast; isolation of infected individuals in one of the special lazarets, or isolation camps, located on the fringes of uninfected zones; the regrouping and re-siting of African populations as part of the overall programme with which the Belgians hoped simultaneously to solve public health, political and economic problems; and, finally, a score of administrative measures designed to regulate various African activities in order to control the incidence and spread of sleeping sickness.

Disease was regarded as an enemy agent against which the Belgian colonial administration fought on these two fronts. The predominantly military administration of the Congo Free State, which was only gradually altered after Leopold's state became a Belgian colony in 1908, quite naturally conceptualised the battle against sleeping sickness as a military campaign, *la lutte*. Sleeping sickness, the foe, had to be isolated, cordoned off, contained and eliminated. After 1903–4 when the aetiology of the disease was discovered, those factors believed by the Europeans to cause the disease – trypanosomes and tsetse-flies – could be targeted for the attack. Supported by the assumption that European science with its superior technology and medicine would succeed where primitive African societies simply floundered, the colonial authorities had no doubts about their methods. After all, said a medical administrator in 1943, 'we know how primitive and futile was the knowledge of the natives in matters of hygiene'.[4]

Diseases, like recalcitrant Africans, were to be forced into submission. In protecting from infection their future labourers and tax-payers, the new colonial authorities felt fully justified in attempting to assert total control. The major feature of the early campaign against sleeping sickness, the *cordon sanitaire*, reflected the paternalistic nature of Belgian colonial policy in which health priorities formed a part of the justification for the methods of the social engineer. African societies, like the labouring classes in Europe, had, it was felt, to be controlled for their own protection. There was a crucial difference, however, in the scope of measures possible in a colonial setting, where social control could sometimes be exercised to a degree unimaginable in the metropole. A growing profusion of legislation from both Brussels and Boma, the capital of the Congo, was sanctioned by the judiciary and enforced by the military and the police. At the same time, an evolving medical infrastructure of personnel, facilities and procedures was directed at locating, isolating and dealing with all those infected with the trypanosome.

Cordon sanitaire and isolation: 1903–9

The sleeping sickness campaign began officially on 5 May 1903 when the Vice Governor-General announced that isolation of victims was the 'principal precaution to take in order to check the spread of the disease'. One doctor raised the 'delicate question' of what to do about victims' families. Should they also be isolated? But, he added, considering the 'insouciance and negligence of hygiene of the Africans', how could effective surveillance be achieved? Reminding the Governor-General that during the recent cholera and plague epidemics in Asia Minor and Arabia more than one port in the Mediterranean had become infected in spite of the *cordon sanitaire*, the doctor explained that he feared the Congolese manifested the same 'hatred of all hygiene measures conceived of by Western civilisation' as did the oriental populations, and that would prevent a successful *cordon* being established.[5]

Local officials as well as all religious and philanthropic organisations in the state were instructed to investigate villages in their localities and alert the chiefs of the measures they were to take. These included, naturally, the isolation of victims at a distance from the village and the burning of their huts, as well as the destruction of all the clothing and daily utensils of those who had died of the disease. There were no instructions on how these aims were to be achieved (even when suitable language translators were available), and there was no discussion of the possible relevance of cultural differences between African societies, especially how these affected indigenous ideas of disease management.

In December 1905 the campaign was futher systematised when formal directions were issued to all colonial agents. Infected individuals were strictly forbidden to travel *except* to lazarets on the instructions of a doctor. Anyone, it was believed, could easily recognise the enlarged glands, particularly the cervical glands at the back of the neck, which were considered to be the main symptom of infection. Agents were accordingly instructed to send suspected victims immediately to the nearest medical post where lymph fluid and blood could be examined under a microscope for evidence of infection. However, under *no* circumstances was a suspect to be sent to an uncontaminated region. If victims had to use river transport, to reach a lazaret, 'they were [to be] placed in movable cages surrounded on all sides by fine wire net' in order to prevent tsetse-flies biting them and spreading the disease.[16]

There were no significant policy changes between 1903 and mid-1906 because there was no available cure and, as sleeping sickness was always fatal, the only feasible measure was the total isolation of all suspected victims. But the situation was greatly changed in December 1906 when new sleeping sickness regulations were issued as a result of the development of the arsenical compound, atoxyl. This drug was valuable for victims in the first stage of the disease while parasites were present in the peripheral circulatory system. It was mistakenly believed that it could effect a cure in four to six weeks, thus regular screening was undertaken to identify suspect cases. Some doctors, however, were reluctant to use atoxyl which they considered to be dangerous even in the hands of specialists.[7]

Surveillance and search

From 1906 the emphasis accordingly shifted to use of the new drug. 'Incessant surveillance' with the full co-operation of all Europeans was henceforth the battle cry of the campaign. Identifying victims in the advanced stages of the disease was not as difficult as the new priority of finding those in the early stages of infection. The latter were both more contagious and, it was believed, more easily curable. Efforts were made to teach African authorities how to look for suspect glands and they were told to report suspected cases immediately. It was deemed imperative that Africans understood the role of the tsetse-fly in spreading the infection and administrators were directed to identify the flies and to convince the chiefs of the importance of clearing away from their villages all tsetse-sheltering bush.[8]

Some state doctors questioned the utility of the policy of isolation as a blanket measure. As one doctor in 1905 explained, there were so many Africans with enlarged glands that isolation of all of them would not only be impossible because of the lack of personnel, it would also paralyse commerce. In his view, 'one could not sequester people without clinical symptoms' other than enlarged glands. He had further doubts about the ethic of infringing upon individual liberty by such a sweeping policy. After all, he pointed out, in Europe, individuals with infectious tuberculosis were allowed to retain their liberty even when the public at large was at risk from infection.[9]

Other doctors were also concerned about the legality of treating patients against their wills. Responding to the queries of a state doctor in 1907, the Director of Justice put the state firmly behind forced treatment, though with some reservations. He declared that the state had not only the right, but even the obligation, to take measures necessary to prevent the spread of contagious and infectious disease. He argued that it was desirable to respect individual liberty as much as possible, but it was the state, not private individuals, which had to take decisions on the best means of fighting an epidemic. This was true even in countries that guaranteed constitutional rights where the individual was sacrificed to the requirements of public security or public hygiene. However, on the question of the right of the state to impose a treatment which sometimes resulted in blindness, the Director of Justice believed that such a therapy would be inhumane and its administration to unwilling victims would be contrary to elementary principles of 'natural law'. If it were proved that such blinding resulted to all those who received it, then it could be used only with the consent of the victim who would have to be forewarned of its danger.[10]

The cordoned 'triangle'

Perhaps the most significant feature of the act of 5 December 1906 was the *cordon sanitaire* it placed around Uele District in the northern Congo, a territory some 300,000 square kilometres in extent. This was achieved by means of a series of lazarets located on the periphery of the district. Between 1907 and 1910 the key lazarets and observation posts were established at the state posts of Ibembo, Barumbu, Stanleyville, Aba and Yakoma. By 1912, there were fourteen observation posts throughout the whole colony, with the major epidemic areas designated as the Semliki basin, Kivu, the Kwilu basin, and Kwango, all lying to the south and west of Province Orientale.[11]

The main principles of the lazaret system were described by Inge Heiberg, the first director of the principal lazaret for the north, located at Ibembo. He advised that isolation camps should be located at the limits of contaminated areas, rather than inside them, and stressed that the traffic caused by labour recruitment from infected areas was highly instrumental in the spread of the disease. All recruitment should be accompanied by thorough medical examinations which should be repeated along the transit routes, and, in effect, constitute a 'sieve' to catch sleeping sickness victims. Heiberg also described how a search tour should be conducted to trap all suspects. The doctor should begin at a point furthest from the centre of the area and in that way 'brush ahead of him like the hunter' all suspects and expel them through the observation post, or 'key' to the district.

Once inside the lazaret, victims would receive atoxyl injections and periodic examinations which were to be carefully recorded in registers. Isolation would vary from complete 'lock-up' to relatively unrestrained surveillance. Heiberg felt that prison-style confinement was administratively preferable for both Europeans and Africans. The boundaries and tasks were clear and public order was not disrupted, 'except, perhaps, at the moment of internment of a sleeping sickness victim'. No meeting could occur between victim and African soldiers or natives and more significantly, no arms would find their way inside the lazaret. 'After all,' the doctor added, 'it is isolation which makes a lazaret.' He saw, however, some disadvantages to the prison-style system, which required, 'energetic and firm surveillance' and other stringent measures. The major problem was the ever-present threat of rebellion, and Heiberg consequently favoured more liberal and open lazarets, keeping strict isolation for the really obstinate or advanced cases.

Patients' families were not officially allowed to visit them in the lazarets, but kin often accompanied victims and tried to remain with them. The conflict which arose from the Belgians' failure to understand the importance of this social aspect of African responses to sickness and disease management provides a rich area of enquiry for the historian.[12] In the early Congo, administrators all too frequently revealed their ignorance of African social and medical practices. But sometimes humanitarian concern broke through, as in 1907 when an unusually sensitive zone administrator addressed the Governor-General: 'I want to know if the families of the patients can live at the post and if they can be rationed by the State, as often, if one member is hospitalized, the others in the family do not want to leave. It would be cruel to send them away.'[13]

The problem of accompanying kin also illuminates the Belgians' extremely legalistic approach to 'native affairs'. For instance, the doctor at Stanleyville lazaret in 1907 asked if he should return the *legitimate* wives of victims to their home villages, pointing out that this would be done only after ascertaining the legality of the marriages, and only one wife would be considered as having legal status.

Heiberg warned that it was of paramount importance to treat the patients with kindness, goodwill and indulgence. They must be carefully fed. He advised that it was best to allow people to live in culturally similar, small groups – 'village style' – with a former sergeant or corporal of the *Force Publique* appointed as the headman. Doctors and administrators should interfere as little as possible in the people's internal disputes.[14]

Lazarets in trouble

By 1910 the prison-style, total isolation system was clearly in difficulties although serious problems had arisen almost immediately with the policy of 1905–6. Lazaret doctors very soon realised that, contrary to earlier hopes, atoxyl cured very few patients in the early stages of the disease, with some relapses, while it had no effect on those in the advanced stages. Africans were very quick to observe the poor results, The mortality rates were appalling – at Ibembo lazaret, nearly one-third of those admitted had died by 1911. Furthermore, there was a dreadful side effect of atoxyl injections – up to thirty per cent of those treated became blind as the drug atrophied the optic nerve. Africans were terrified of *la lutte* and the lazarets became popularly known as 'death camps'. Wild rumours circulated that the colonial officials were not only causing the disease, but were rounding up people in order to eat them. A missionary's advice of 1902 that the state should establish 'colonies of incurables' had been made a reality.[15]

Heiberg's professional experience in European insane asylums makes it most relevant to note his views on the difference between an insane European and an African sleeping sickness patient. According to him, nearly all European patients in an asylum would have their own particular delusions. That made a co-ordinated riot in a hospital an unknown, even impossible event. But in the Congo, thought Heiberg, sleeping sickness victims had a different kind of 'insanity'. Their disease reduced, but did not destroy, their power to reason. Sleeping sickness victims were obsessed with such ideas as 'the injustice of their imprisonment', and a hundred sleeping sickness victims with an identical 'obsession' comprised a formidable threat. When the local administrator visited the lazaret in September 1910, he was repeatedly approached by patients with the same complaint that they were being prevented from 'seeing home'.

Heiberg's views on insane and 'irrational' behaviour are of interest in that they reveal contemporary European attitudes about the insane as obsessive people who have fixed ideas and who act individually, not in groups. Among Africans, however, Heiberg proposed a different kind of insanity, that of a group of people sharing an obsessive and irrational idea. Perhaps more importantly, he could only view the Africans' desire to escape western biomedicine in order to return to their own people and their ways of dealing with misfortune as totally irrational – or insane – behaviour. Like many colonialists, he believed that Africans were acting irrationally in rejecting the benefits of western civilisation.[16]

All along, some lazaret inmates had managed to escape into the surrounding areas, but the growing frustration and hostility of the victims isolated at Ibembo found expression in two serious riots in 1909 and 1910, thus confirming Heiberg's concerns. The Ibembo riots signalled the need for reform. As Heiberg said of the lazaret in 1910, 'Strictly speaking, it was a permanent prison and should bear the inscription, "Abandon all hope, ye who enter here."'[17]

The sleeping sickness campaign, like other Belgian colonial policies, was highly centralised with most instructions issued directly from Brussels. There was no separate colonial medical department until December 1922. A medical service had functioned from Brussels since December 1909, but doctors in the colony remained strictly subordinated to the authority of their local territorial administrators. Before December 1910 and the first medical department for the Congo, there was no true 'medical authority which made sanitation regulations'. All such regulations were issued by civil and military authorities. Thus measures such as medical passports and the epidemiological maps upon which the *cordon sanitaire* was based emanated from non-medical administrators. Ordinances controlling African life – village siting, fishing, salt-production, travel, kin relations – were all drafted by non-medical staff.

At the same time, doctors who were instructed to carry out the sleeping sickness measures frequently found themselves in the impossible situation of having to request assistance from the local territorial administrator. And, very often, the administrator was reluctant to support the doctors' requests. The main reason for the lack of co-operation was the political necessity of maintaining African tolerance for Belgian rule. Implementing public health measures made the local administrator more unpopular that he already was among the people. Pressed to achieve certain political and economic goals, namely labour recruitment and tax collection, the local administrators chose to ignore medical and public health measures as much as they could.

In 1909 the major features of *la lutte* were the *cordon sanitaire* and isolation in lazarets, considered by one doctor as being together 'the great panacea for public health in the Congo'. But, as he acknowledged, combined with the ineffective, even dangerous, chemotherapy, the campaign evoked intense distrust from the people. Furthermore, he said, the sporadic surveys for victims in African villages were viewed as 'little more than man hunts' and the result was that 'people fled [from] the doctors more quickly than they did the tax collectors!'[18] Often the army was required to assist doctors to examine Africans and then to effect their isolation. Clearly, the combination of a complicated and blundering bureaucracy with an isolation system from which the only exit was escape or death and in which one third of those treated became blind was a failure.

African responses to the early period of *la lutte* made it apparent to the colonial administration that no public health programme could be really effective unless everyone involved, African and European, co-operated. Slowly, the realisation dawned that medical and administrative staff would have to co-operate in order to implement sleeping sickness measures. There had been calls previously for the understanding and support of African authorities in the campaign to examine all of the people and to isolate infected individuals, but by late 1909 it had become clear that the understanding and support of all Africans affected by the campaign would be necessary if it were to stand any chance of success. The responses of the people to the Belgian sleeping sickness campaign were indeed a significant factor which shaped the future development of public health in the colony.

The pre-war period: 1910–1914

There were significant reforms in both health policy and the colonial medical service in the years immediately preceding the First World War. The shift began in 1910 with a series of reforms. The major change in policy was that lazarets were to be more open, becoming 'village-lazarets' in which only very advanced or troublesome patients would stay. Unlike the prison-like atmosphere of the earlier lazarets, the new institutions would accommodate members of the victims' immediate families. All other victims of the disease would be treated as out-patients and attend injection clinics which would be conveniently located near their own homes. Thus victims, while still able to do so, could continue labouring or being involved in food production.[19]

The reforms reflected administrative concerns beyond purely medical ones, and several issues were involved. First, there was the serious matter of the notorious reputation of the Leopoldian administration of the Congo Free State which the Belgian government wished to dispel after it took over in 1908. Then, too, the Belgians were still greatly involved in the process of establishing state control in several parts of the Congo including the northeast. Thus, while still engaged in the process of conquest and consolidating, the administration of the new colony had to appear to be more humane than Leopold's regime in order to avoid further condemnation by the 'Great Powers'.

While it is important to see events during this period in the context of the broader political policy of improving the administration's image, it must be pointed out that medical personnel in the Congo had been lobbying for some time for the creation of a separate medical department which would permit the rationalisation of the health service and enable the development of a more systematic public health policy. Following a tour of a district much infected with sleeping sickness, the Governor-General in 1910 proposed a major new campaign to combat the disease throughout the colony. The combination of pressure from colonial doctors for a medical department and the apparently increasing epidemicity of sleeping sickness resulted in the creation of such a department at the end of 1909, although a comprehensive sleeping sickness programme was not put into effect until 1918. The new medical department, like other branches of the colonial administration, was still based in Belgium where it remained so firmly centralised that one contemporary commented that the sleeping sickness campaign was being fought from offices in Brussels, not Africa.[20]

Sleeping sickness and administrative control

Sleeping sickness policy was intertwined with broader issues of territorial administration, and this linkage began to emerge clearly after 1910. For instance, there was the problem of controlling the movements of people both within the colony and across its international frontiers. French Congo, Sudan and Uganda, all bordering the north-east, each contained areas of seriously epidemic sleeping sickness by 1910. The movements of people in and out of the Congo was therefore a primary concern for the administration. There was significant interplay between sleeping sickness measures, particularly those concerning the *cordon sanitaire*, and the broader economic and social concerns of territorial administration. Northern Congo was an important source of labour for economic projects such as the Kilo-Moto Gold Mines, the army and road construction. Those responsible for labour recruitment for these activities pressured the colonial authorities to allow easy access to African labour in the northern Congo while at the same time the medical experts pressed for stricter controls over population movements in order to protect the northern Congo from sleeping sickness. Ironically, one colonial sector, the economic, pushed for policies which could adversely affect the health of Africans while another colonial sector, the medical, strove to protect Africans from the spread of disease. Colonial policy was not monolithic but was instead a combination of interests which sometimes conflicted. It would be farfetched to impute Machiavellian motives to those who made public health policy and to the local administrators who implemented measures. Nevertheless, sleeping sickness measures formed part of the system of control used by the Belgian rulers.

The crucial element in the reform of sleeping sickness policy was the introduction on 30 April 1910 of mandatory medical passports.[21] Formerly, all Africans travelling beyond the immediate confines of their home regions had been required to obtain a travel pass on which doctors recorded details of all medical examinations. From April 1910 the new medical passports superseded the less-specific travel documents in the increasing attempt to control every movement of Africans.

An important element in the revision of public health policy was the standardisation of observation posts. These were strategically located surveillance and screening stations at which a medical helper, ideally a European *agent sanitaire*, or medical assistant, but very often a lone African *infirmier*, or dresser, was based with a microscope. It was his duty to screen all travellers, being especially alert to those coming from regions known to be infected with the disease. A major function of the observation post was issuing medical passports in an attempt to further restrict movements of people.

It had been said that considering the large numbers of victims and restricted resources and personnel, that much of the voluminous legislation was 'of academic interest' only, a mere 'paper war'. While it is true that many of the instructions could not be successfully implemented because of the lack of resources, especially personnel, it would be a mistake to dismiss the early sleeping sickness policy as simply a 'paper war'. Many state officials ignored the regulations, but others made considerable effort to enforce them.[23]

Another significant feature of the campaign in this early period was the emergence of a discernible policy regarding the organisation and shape of African societies. Re-structuring African societies would remain for decades an important and troublesome issue for the colonial authorities. It became a particular problem when the public health authorities came into conflict with the local administrators, for the two departments had quite different motives for wishing to reorganise African society. When the two were in agreement over the reorganisation and re-siting of a group of people, there was less conflict, although increasingly, territorial administrators were loathe to involve themselves in a form of administrative interference which was so unpopular with the people.

From very early in the campaign against sleeping sickness, the regrouping and relocation of African populations had been a much used tactic. Ostensibly to protect people from the danger of infection through proximity to the infected tsetse-flies, the regrouping and relocation of entire populations also conveniently served other requirements of the local administration, especially during the early colonial period when state control was still precarious. Local administrators preferred their subjects to be sited for ease of administrative access even though many agents actually on the scene were extremely reluctant to tamper with this aspect of African life for fear of increased hostility and resistance. This tactic was important in labour recruitment and tax collection. It was simply easier to deal with groups of people conveniently located near communication routes or administrative centres than it was to 'chase up' scattered individuals far from the main sites of colonial power. With some people like the Azande, whose normal settlement pattern was one of dispersed family clusters separated by stretches of forest or savannah, the policy of regrouping was especially controversial. The topography of most of the northern Congo made it impractical to attempt to relocate Africans away from tsetse areas, and when such moves were carried out, people simply returned to their rivers to fish and to their fields to cultivate. During this early period of the campaign it was quite unrealistic for the colonial authorities to think of a grand restructuring of African socieities, if for no other reason than the lack of staff and resources to enforce such policy. Nevertheless, it was often discussed, and it was an important underlying consideration behind sleeping sickness policy.[25]

By 1910, doctors had been delegated considerable powers by the central administration in Belgium to request the reorganisation and relocation of Africans within their districts. Also by 1910, doctors had the right to request assistance from the army – the *force publique* – as well as the co-operation of the territorial administration, in their attempts to implement the public health policy. Thus it was not uncommon for the doctor to arrive in an area accompanied by armed soldiers and an administrator, and then to begin a systematic examination of the people, who were obliged by this show of force to present themselves regardless of the activities they may have been engaged in at the time. The doctor was also entitled to the co-operation of the local *capitas*, or village headmen appointed by the state, as well as that of the *chef médaille*, or officially recognised chief, also a colonial appointment. But these were not the only authority figures available to implement the programme. From 1912 most posts had, in addition to their contingent of the *force publique*, other law enforcement agents in the form of police who might be territorial or local. Finally, by 1912, the central government had made it quite clear that every European in the district – whether in government employment or not – was obliged to participate in the campaign against sleeping sickness.[26]

The First World War

The exigencies of war revealed not only the coercive nature of European medical intervention in the Belgian Congo, they also brought about changes in the nature of that intervention. An outstanding feature of the sleeping sickness campaign during the First World War was the manner in which the colonial administration contradicted its own public health policy and, in fact, in so doing aggravated the problem of human sleeping sickness in the northern Congo. The war meant that the Belgian government needed the labour and resources available in its colony more than ever before. Evacuated to England because of the German occupation of Belgium, the Belgian government looked to its African colony for material assistance in the war effort and the northern Congo was suddenly of great importance as the provider of three vital resources – gold, rubber and men.

But the increasing demands for gold, rubber and labour forced the colonial administration to violate much of its own recent public health policy in the northeast. The escalating labour requirements resulted in an intensification of the movement of population throughout the northeast, and thus the recently imposed *cordon sanitaire* became a hindrance to the war effort. Until the early 1920s both rubber and gold production remained particularly labour-intensive activities which required substantial investment of production forces.[27]

It is clear from the evidence that, at the local and provincial levels, administrators in the northern Congo were anxious to continue the campaign against sleeping sickness during the war. In spite of growing evidence that there were areas of epidemic sleeping sickness in north-central Uele, the Belgian administration remained unwilling to acknowledge the local government's claims that such regions were epidemic because it wished to avoid the restrictions of an effective *cordon sanitaire*. The war further exacerbated such differences of opinion. Unfortunately for the inhabitants, it was precisely the north-central regions of Uele district that were richest in wild rubber and Africans were continually pressured by the state to collect rubber to meet their tax demands. The rubber was most prolific in tsetse-infested gallery forests where trees and brush grew fringe-like along the waterways. It was quite clear, complained the District Commissioner, that the central government simply refused to declare an epidemic in north-central Uele district and such official recognition was required before a *cordon sanitaire* could be legally enforced. As a result, during the First World War there was a slow-down, virtually a cessation, of the campaign to control sleeping sickness in the northern Congo.

A major consequence of the war for Uelians was the increase and spread of epidemic sleeping sickness.[28] In some north-central territories like Gwane, Bili and Dakwa where the disease was already serious, sleeping sickness now became intensely epidemic with entire *chefferies* afflicted. The region would have to await the end of the war before the first really effective steps were taken to cope with the increase and spread of the disease – the first effective steps, that is, from the point of view of the 'medicalisation' of the region.

Missions maladie du sommeil: 1920–30

> The most highly organised attempts to deal with the problems of endemic disease were the mobile services set up in Africa to combat human trypanosomiasis and on to these were later grafted field units with wider terms of reference, whose diagnostic and treatment facilities

were directed at a number of different endemic disease problems.[29]

During the decade 1920–30 special sleeping sickness missions were launched and developed. For many Congolese, these teams were their first intimate contact with the new colonial state. It was a contact not always comprehensible or pleasant. *Missions maladie du sommeil* were special teams which were systematically to survey certain regions of the colony in order to identify and treat victims in their own villages. The cardinal features of the teams were their mobility and their attempt to examine the entire African population of the colony. New staff was recruited specifically for this campaign, and the hope of the Governor-General who first ennunciated the programme in August 1917 was that the colonial medical service would be able to recruit medical staff in Europe when military corps began demobilising following the end of the war.[30]

The first sleeping sickness team in the Belgian Congo began functioning in Kwango District in 1919, followed by a second team in Uele in 1920. Within four years three more sleeping sickness teams were established in Bangala, Stanleyville and Mayumbe districts. So well did this policy take hold that by 1932 there were at least five such teams operating in the northeast alone: Uele, Semliki, Stanleyville-Basoko, Kivu, and Maniema. But difficulties soon emerged. The divergent goals of different colonial departments resulted in *impasses* over the implementation of the public health measures. Doctors found themselves confronted with local administrators who were unwilling to enforce public health policies and recommendations. In addition, increasingly through the 1920s, the work and responsibilities of the special sleeping sickness teams overlapped with the colonial medical service until it became very difficult to perceive separate and distinctive roles for the two services.

The surveys continued almost annually between 1920 and 1930. Basically, the aim was the identification and treatment of every single victim in the colony, an ambitious goal indeed. It was not always easy to gain the co-operation of the people, and thus the colonial doctors often found it useful to be accompanied by the local headman who was familiar with the territory and who could locate the isolated settlements. It was also found useful to take along police agents who could assist with 'recalcitrants' and those who attempted to flee.

All adult males in the *chefferies* were given identity cards which displayed the names of their wives and children, and the sleeping sickness team issued dated medical visas with details of their examinations. The most important individual who helped with the survey, according to one survey director, was the chief, and if he happened to be co-operative the number of daily examinations was greatly increased. For instance, people working in the fields were most reluctant to break off to attend medical examinations and were only brought in with difficulty. Here the chief's persuasion could be vital. Some groups, like the Azande, always hid their women from the teams. Although ambulatory patients were supposed to present themselves for fortnightly injections, it was 'extremely rare' for patients to appear voluntarily fortnightly or even monthly. One doctor voiced the ceaseless complaint of the coloniser, 'We do not know how to change African thinking.'[31]

Settlement patterns: social engineering and medical missions

By 1931 the sleeping sickness campaign reflected both major strands of Belgian public health policy – *prophylaxie médicale* and *prophylaxie biologique.* It was in the latter, the realm of 'social engineering', that colonial doctors were most often frustrated, especially as they found themselves in the awkward situation of making demands which conflicted with the goals of other sectors of the colonial administration.

There was a serious lack of co-ordination, and even conflict, between various administrative departments in the colony according to Marone, the doctor in charge of the 1931 survey. He urged that doctors be granted sanctions to arm them in their attempts to effect reorganisation of African societies for the purposes of public health as this remained the greatest problem facing the sleeping sickness campaign. He devoted fifteen pages of his 1931 report to a discussion of the one issue of regrouping and re-siting of Africans. Since clearing all of the tsetse-infested brush along major rivers was impossible, it was particularly important, he felt, to reorganise people into villages which should be placed at locations 'chosen by the medical service' in accord with the territorial administration. As things were, he said, doctors could only attempt medical prophylaxis: biological prophylaxis, the 'social engineering', was up to the territorial administration. Clearly severe tensions had developed between medical staff, who pressed for further preventive measures, and local administrators, who saw medicine as limited to a curative function.

Marone's lengthy articulation of the frustration experienced by doctors in their attempts to advise and implement public health measures designed to prevent the spread of the disease, reveals the extent of this problem by 1930. From 1920, doctors had implored territorial administrators to heed certain measures which, they believed, would decrease the incidence of sleeping sickness. The measures focused on several critical areas of African life including population movements due to their own travel, labour recruitment, kin ties and trade. Doctors were concerned about the movements of Africans induced by their search for rubber, and the medical authorities expressed reservations about the epidemiologically deleterious effects of state taxation policies. They offered advice on matters concerning African economic activities such as fishing and trade. They advised the 'sealing off' of certain badly afflicted regions, asking that outsiders be prevented entry even when seeking to fulfil their mandatory rubber tax. Medical advice related to sleeping sickness touched upon state policies concerning the growing of cash crops such as cotton, and those concerning porterage and road construction were directly affected by the acceptance of such medical advice. By 1930 the issue of regrouping people into larger villages and resiting villages in areas considered safer from infection of sleeping sickness had become a major problem for the medical staff and for the local administration alike.

From the mid-1920s, demands by some doctors for greater autonomy for the special sleeping sickness teams conflicted with the demands of others who recommended unification of the two services. Discrete sleeping sickness teams functioned alongside an evolving colonial medical service, but there was considerable confusion as the two services tended to compete for the same limited funds and personnel. Resources were shunted between the two services, producing uncertainty over which staff or facilities belonged to which service and which functions were the responsibility of each.

The relation of the sleeping sickness missions to the medical service became more, rather than less, unclear over time. In 1924 Dr Van Campenhout, the director of the *Service de l'Hygiène* at the Colonial Ministry in Brussels and a man who just two years earlier had solidly supported the special sleeping sickness team concept, suggested that the autonomous sleeping sickness teams be discontinued. He felt that one single, unified colonial medical service could better manage the sleeping sickness campaign.[32] By 1928 the chief medical officer felt that the sleeping sickness mission had 'lost sight of its principal aim', which was the survey of the district for all victims of the disease; instead it had become 'bogged down' in the treatment of victims. The head of the provincial medical service in Province Orientale thought that the same goals could be attained with half the staff if redundancies were

E

eliminated: 'I have not been able to find a clear line of demarcation between the work of the regular Medical Service and the Sleeping Sickness Mission of Uele. The latter spends a great deal of its effort on "general medicine".'

Some doctors were 'too busy with private patients'. Dispensaries directed by the district medical service were next door to dispensaries, and in one case, to a hospital, directed by the chief of the sleeping sickness team. Throughout the decade the confusion increased between the roles of the sleeping sickness missions and those of the medical service until by the end of the 1920s the medical tactics, too, were being challenged with explicit complaints about the system's 'creaking bureaucracy'.[33]

By 1930, *la lutte* reached into every area of life for both coloniser and colonised in the northern Congo, and had become inextricably entangled with other sectors of the colonial administration. Measures advised by medical authorities to curb the spread of sleeping sickness unavoidably affected areas of colonial policy such as transport, road construction and villagisation. African life, too, was markedly affected by the public health measures that had been instituted.

Summary

Events in the northern Congo between 1903 and 1930 are illustrative of the ways in which disease, especially when epidemic, can both illuminate social relations and itself affect the course of history. Medicine clearly helped to shape the political and administrative character of imperialism in the early Belgian Congo. Government responses to epidemic sleeping sickness in the Congo were at first predominantly legislative while the colonial medical service and a sleeping sickness campaign only gradually took shape. The pervasive, bureaucratic nature of Belgian colonial policy was exemplified in public health and medicine too, with local administrators being inundated with instructions, ordinances and decrees concerning sleeping sickness policies. These also touched upon myriad aspects of African life and by their very complexity led to confusion in the actual implementation of medical policy, while administrative neglect of medical requirements led to conflict with the political and economic ambitions of colonial officialdom.

Notes

1 Ministère des Affaires Etrangères, Archives Africaines, Brussels. [Hereafter MAEAA] MAEAA 4389.1090, 19 November 1943, Dr A. Duren to Leemans, des Distributions d'Eau, Brussels, 'Etat sanitaire des populations du Congo avant sa colonisation par la Belgique.'

2 D. J. Bradley, 'The situation and the response', in E. E. Sabben-Clare, K. Kirkwood and D. J. Bradley, *Health in Tropical Africa During the Colonial Period.* Oxford, 1980, p. 9.

3 F. M. J. C. Nevens, 'Projet de plan général de l'organisation de la lutte contre les trypanosomiases en Afrique', *Bulletin de la Académie Royale des Sciences d'Outre-Mer,* Classes des Sciences Naturelles et Médicales, XVII, 1965, pp. 12-13.

4 MAEAA 4389.1090, 19 November 1943, Duren to Leemans.

5 MAEAA 846.18, 22 February 1903, Secretary of State to Governor-General; MAEAA 846.19, 4 April 1903, Broden to Governor-General.

6 Musée Royal de l'Afrique Centrale, Section Historique, Archives, Tervuren, Belgium. [Hereafter MRAC] Fuchs papers 114, 7 December 1905, Vice-Governor Lantonnois to all administrators, camp commanders, doctors, missionaries and companies.

7 J. Rodhain, 'Documents pour servir à l'histoire de la maladie du sommeil au Congo Belge, III. La période 1907 à 1911. Les premiers lazarets et les débuts de l'expérimentation de l'atoxyl et de l'émétique', *Bulletin de l'Institut Royal Colonial Belge,* XIX, 1948, pp. 943-55; F. M. J. C. Nevens, 'Projet de plan général de l'organisation de la lutte contre les trypanosomiases en Afrique', p. 11. MAEAA 847.372, 25 January 1908, Dr Zerbini; MAEAA 838.3, 19 June 1908, Vice Governor-General to Secretary of State.

8 MRAC 50.30.221, 16 October 1912, Chef de Zone André Landeghem to all Administrateurs Territoriales.

9 MAEAA 847.112, 28 November 1905, Dr Zerbini, Boma to Governor-General.

10 MAEAA 845.6, 24 October 1907, Director of Justice, de Meulemeester to Director of the Medical Service; 4 September 1907, Note for Governor-General.

11 MAEAA 4420.20, 25 September 1912, Notes for the 1913 Annual Report.

12 J. M. Janzen with Dr Arkinstall, *The Quest for Therapy in Lower Zaire,* Berkeley, 1978, pp. 3-11.

13 MAEAA 843.1, 19 July 1907, Landeghem to Governor-General.

14 MAEAA 843.20, 14 February 1910, Dr Heiberg, Report on Ibembo Lazaret; MRAC Fuchs Papers 114, Dr Trolli 1907; MAEAA 843.35, 29 September 1910, Landeghem to Governor-General.

15 J. Rodhain, 'Documents pour servir à l'histoire de la maladie du sommeil au Congo Belge, III. La période 1907 à 1911. Les premiers lazarets et les débuts de l'expérimentation de l'atoxyl et de l'émétique', *Bulletin de l'Institut Royal Colonial Belge,* XIX, 1948, p. 950; J. Schwetz, *L'Evolution de la Médecine au Congo Belge,* p. 100. Schwetz reported the rumour widespread among Africans that the sick were inoculated with the illness by the Europeans who then placed them inside lazarets to await their deaths. The bodies, it was believed, were then 'cut into bits and put into containers sold in the shops under the names "corned beef", "carbonnade flammands", etc.' MAEAA 846.1, 24 October 1902, Dr Rossignon to Governor-General.

16 MAEAA 843.20, 14 February 1910, Heiberg Report; MAEAA 843.35, 29 September 1910, Chef de Zone Landeghem to Governor-General; MAEAA 843.20, 14 February 1910.

17 MAEAA 843.20, 14 February 1910, Heiberg Report.

18 MAEAA 4419.4, c. 1909; J. Rodhain, 'Notes et propositions'; Schwetz: 'l'Evolution de la Médecine au Congo Belge, p. 90.

19 MAEAA 4419.602, 25 June 1909, A. Broden to Minister enclosing 'La lutte contre la trypanose humaine,' by Doctors Broden and Rodhain; MAEAA 843.20, 14 February 1910, Heiberg Report; MAEAA 847.143, 23 April 1906, J. Todd to Van Campenhout.

20 MAEAA 850.9, 10 May 1918, Governor-General to all Vice Governor-Generals and District Commissioners; F. O. Stohr in *Bulletin of the Sleeping Sickness Bureau*, 4, 1912, p. 302.

21 MAEAA 850.260, 30 April 1910, Vice Governor-General Fuchs' circular.

22 MAEAA 847.143, 23 April 1906, J. L. Todd to Van Campenhout; MAEAA 831, 10 June 1910, *Mesures complementaires prises en 1910 pour enrayer le developpement de la maladie du sommeil*; MAEAA 848.114, 17 January 1910; MAEAA 848.115, 17 January 1910; MAEAA 849.206, 30 April 1910, Fuchs' instruction on medical passports; 8 September 1910, *Receuil Mensuel*, 9 (new sleeping sickness regulations which replaced those of 5 December 1906).

23 On Paper War, see J. Burke, 'Historique de la lutte contre la maladie du sommeil au Congo'. *Annales de la Société Belge de Médecine*, 51, 1971, p. 468. For instance in 1911, the doctor at Buta complained that issuing medical passports took up half of each day. MAEAA 849.291, 18 May 1911.

24 MAEAA Affaires Indigènes, 1422.3, 27 August 1929, Gregoire, 'Rapport politique, 1929, District de l'Uele-Nepoko.' MAEAA Rapports Congo Belge 151.1, 21 May 1932, Dr L. Fontana.

25 MAEAA 4429.20, 25 September 1912, Note for 1913 annual report of the medical service.

26 MAEAA 848.118, 29 October 1909. For instance, Dr Heiberg suggested to the Governor-General that special 'sanitary police' should be based at Aba and frequently patrol the frontier.

27 MRAC 50.30.16, Landeghem, 'Rapport Annuel, Bas-Uele, 1915'. MRAC 50.30.156, 23 July 1915, Vice Governor-General Malfeyt. Circular to administrators in Province Orientale.

28 MRAC 50.30.91, 19 September 1915, Dr Dubois, Buta to District Commissioner, Buta.

29 A. J. Duggan, 'Tropical medicine: a submerging art?', *Transactions of the Royal Society of Tropical Hygiene and Medicine*, 76, 1982, p. 569.

30 MAEAA 850.9, 10 May 1918, Governor-General to Vice Governor-General and District Commissioners. These ideas parallel those implemented in neighbouring French territories a year earlier. In 1916, the French Colonel Jamot had created the first *equipes mobiles* to survey and treat sleeping sickness in the Oubangui-Chari region of French Congo. It was a new idea of 'mobile-prevention'. Marcel Beby Eyidi, *Le Vainqueur de la Maladie du Sommeil: le Docteur Eugène Jamot, 1879–1937*, Paris, 1950, p. 45.

31 MAEAA 855.63, 18 November 1921, Dr S'Heeren Report of Sleeping Sickness Mission in Uele District.

32 MAEAA 4461.56, 3 September 1924, Emile Van Campenhout, London, 'Report to the Société des Nations, Re: Campagne contre la maladie du sommeil en Afrique équatoriale.'

33 MAEAA Rapports Congo Belge 150.1, 12 April 1929, J. Schwetz, Report on Sleeping Sickness in Province Orientale.

CHAPTER SIX

Cholera and the origins of the American sanitary order in the Philippines

Reynaldo C. Ileto

Even nationalist writers in the Philippines find it impossible to interrogate the established notion that among the blessings of American colonial rule was a sanitary regime which saved countless Filipino lives. Take the historians T. A. Agoncillo and M. C. Guerrero. In their influential textbook they narrate in some detail the Philippine-American war of 1899–1902, highlighting the Filipino struggle to defend their independence 'through blood and tears'. In marked contrast to colonial historians, they stress that although the republican commander-in-chief Emilio Aguinaldo had been captured in mid-1901, guerrilla warfare continued under the leadership of General Miguel Malvar until relentless American campaigns forced him to surrender on 16 April 1902.

Agoncillo and Guerrero uphold their anti-colonial stance in the discussion, several chapters later, of the educational system ('originally established as an instrument of pacification'). But upon reaching the topic of health and welfare, they seem to switch to another register:

> Before 1900, ravages of cholera, smallpox, dysentery, malaria, tuberculosis, and other deadly diseases plagued the people. . . . When the Americans came, they immediately set to work to minimize the spread of diseases and to improve, on the other hand, the health of the people. Epidemics that used to migrate to the Philippines were either prevented or minimized by the establishment of the Quarantine Service supervised by competent American doctors and public health officers.

The distinction between nationalist and colonial writing collapses. The task of educating the people in the 'elementary principles of hygiene and sanitation' was difficult, continue Agoncillo and Guerrero, because the Filipinos were

> superstition-ridden and ignorant of the strange power of the minute

> germs to cause deadly diseases, and were not easily convinced by the efficacy of medical methods in combating the cause of death from various sickness. The early Americans, then, were up against a formidable wall of ignorance and superstition.[1]

The 1899–1902 war of resistance and the 1902–4 cholera epidemic belong to two distinct series in Philippine historiography. The former is a moment in the epic struggle for independence from colonial rule, the latter a Philippine chapter in the saga of scientific progress. Like their nineteenth-century forebear José Rizal – the 'father' of nationalist historiography *and* doctor of medicine – Agoncillo and Guerrero as well as most others of the Filipino intelligentsia order the past in terms of the triumph of reason and science over superstition and backwardness. The apparent victory over the cholera in 1902–3 is thus assimilated into the universal history of medical progress, torn from its original moorings in a colonial war and pacification campaign.

Much of this disjunction stems from the fact that the most accessible accounts of cholera epidemics during the first decade of American rule are authored by the very architects of the anti-cholera measures: the Secretary of the Interior, Dean Worcester, and the Commissioner of Public Health, Dr Victor Heiser.[2] The epidemic, says Worcester, 'came soon after the close of a long continued war', hence not a few 'evil-intentioned persons' took the opportunity to make trouble.[3] Worcester knew that the rumour-mongering and the popular resistance to his cholera campaign formed some continuity with the recent war (which was, in fact, still raging at the time the epidemic struck). However, since the health campaign is represented in purely medico-sanitary terms, and resistance to it conflated with superstition and backwardness, the issue of colonial domination simply fades away.

It is instructive to juxtapose Worcester's representation of the war against cholera, which he himself led, with his eyewitness account of a famous battle between American and Filipino forces in 1899, in which even the American commander praised the courage of the outgunned Filipino soldiers. Worcester could only perceive, and describe, the 'gallant advance' and 'intrepidity' of American troops. He turned the Filipinos, his biographer R. J. Sullivan notes, into 'almost impersonal props in a drama whose theme was American heroism and military skill; if "not retreating in great disorder", or fleeing "in confusion towards Imus" they were presented pictorially, impersonal beings whose very anonymity highlighted American individuality and military skill.'[4]

The fight against the cholera of 1902–4 has been represented, even by nationalist writers, in similar fashion: as a drama whose theme is American heroism and medico-sanitary skill, where Filipino participants – the victims from the poorer classes in particular – function as the anonymous backdrop for the saga of progress. This study attempts to put such claims into question by exploring those months of turmoil in 1902 when the war against the cholera and the 'pacification' of Filipinos were barely differentiated, when medico-sanitary measures and popular resistance to such, were continuing acts of war.

On 14 March 1902, a vessel from Hong Kong arrived in Manila with cholera on its bill of health. Despite strict quarantine inspections and prohibitions on such incoming vessels, shortly afterwards the first cases of cholera were discovered in a barrio called Farola near the mouth of the Pasig river where many stevedores, fishermen and petty smugglers lived.[5] From here spread the epidemic which devasted the country up to November 1902, lingered on till early February 1904, and ultimately claimed a total – conservatively estimated – of 109,461 deaths, 4,386 of which were in Manila.

Upon confirmation of the existence of cholera Secretary Worcester mobilised both civilian and military personnel to contain its spread. The Farola district was razed and its inhabitants moved to a detention camp. The attempt to contain the epidemic in Manila proved fruitless, however, as people managed to 'escape' by night or even by day through the ricefields. Small native canoes carried the infection to the towns around Manila bay. Worcester compared the situation to the U.S. army's attempt, several years earlier, to cordon off Manila from republican forces surrounding it: 'What General Otis could not accomplish with thousands of soldiers was an impossibility for the board of health, aided by the city police and a few hundred men from the insular constabulary.'[6]

The cholera was certainly impossible to contain, for even American troop movements contributed to its spread. A military transport vessel carried it to the city of Nueva Caceres, in the southeastern part of Luzon, 'from which source it was transmitted to a large number of pueblos in that section'.[7] The first cases at Pagsanjan and Majayjay in Laguna province were among two batches of soldiers sent up from Camp Wallace in Manila on 24 April 1902.[8] Cholera was introduced into the Mariquina valley east of Manila by troops sent to guard against infection of the Manila water supply.[9] The board of health in that province warned constabulary detachments to keep out of the towns because they had infected one already.[10]

The cholera swiftly spread up the Pasig river arteries leading to the

Mariquina valley and the coastal towns of (lake) Laguna de Bay, until it arrived upon the terrain of guerrilla resistance to American occupation: the provinces of Laguna, Batangas and Tayabas. In fact, it was the exigencies of war that caused a delay of about a month before the lake towns of Laguna were infected. On 10 December of the previous year all ports had been closed as part of General J. Franklin Bell's all-out effort to force Malvar's capitulation. The cessation of native traffic in the lake severely restricted the flow of supplies to the guerrilla camps, and held back the cholera as well. On 19 April, three days after Malvar's surrender, all restrictions to trade and travel in the region were to be lifted, but the cholera forced the ports to remain closed in order to give time for local health boards to organise and take the required precautions.[11]

As long as the ports remained closed, no cholera appeared, 'but immediately on opening them [on the first of May] the disease attacked first the ports and thence spread back into the country'. The coastal quarantine proved useless as infected Filipinos and 'occasional Americans' managed to land surreptitiously, usually at night between ports. The shallow waters of the lake made it possible for some to wade ashore from quarantined boats up to half a kilometre distant. 'The disease once landed made universal progress, especially through the barrios.'[12]

Cholera claimed its victims from all levels of society, including American soldiers and residents, prominent Filipinos, Chinese, and Spaniards. The distribution of victims among the races and social classes was, however, unequal.[13] Americans, Spaniards and Chinese had well-equipped hospitals catering specially for them. At the Santiago cholera hospital, on the other hand, the vast majority of patients belonged to the 'unintelligent' class, among whom the rate of recovery was as low as 5.32 per cent. This was attributed to bad sanitary conditions and 'poor food in their everyday lives' which produced 'such a low state of vitality that the system was unable to react from effects of the toxin produced by the cholera organisms'.[14] Overcrowding, poor sanitation, and poor diet in certain districts of Manila were the primary causes of the malignancy of the cholera among the lower classes.

In the provinces south and east of Manila where guerrilla resistance had been intense, the epidemic was 'especially severe'.[15] The chief army surgeon noted in mid-June that 'in Laguna, Batangas, and the adjacent part of the province of Tayabas, cholera [had] spread in virulent epidemic form, hundreds of cases probably having occurred without report'.[16] The 'sad and impressive' mortality figures – a recent study put the death toll for Batangas alone at 20,000 – were attributed to the fact that 'both troops and natives had, especially in Batangas and Laguna, been recently subjected to the demoralising and debilitating influences of war'.[17]

War, the cholera, and famine conditions came together, at least in southwestern Luzon. Such connections would be obscured if we relied on reports emanating from Manila. All we have, really, is this note by the Commissioner of Public Health in his report for August: 'In one or two instances it has been necessary to send food, the scarcity of rice existing in some of the towns being so great as to become an important factor in the cholera situation.'[18] Poverty and malnutrition, together with poor sanitation, are mentioned as some of the causes of the 'malignancy' of the epidemic among the lower classes. But any connection with the war is muted. When the concentration camps are mentioned, as in the Surgeon General's report for 1902, it is claimed that people in them had never experienced better living conditions and thus survived the epidemic better.[19]

Let us re-examine those critical months of March to May 1902. According to Malvar, his decision to surrender on 16 April was forced by

> the reconcentration in zones, the extinction of food supplies in the country. . . . If I had not know what was passing with the people who petitioned my surrender that their deaths were very certain in the coming year, 1903, unless they could plant the rice in the month of May, I should not have surrendered.[20]

Malvar must have known, too, that the cholera, then ravaging Manila, was already present in his northernmost zone of operations, Laguna province. The official date of the cholera's first appearance in Laguna is 7 April. Five days later, the U.S. commander at Calamba, the provincial capital, reported a suspected case in a native barge that had arrived from Manila. The following day, a nipa hut was burned in a barrio at the edge of town after its owner's wife had died of cholera.[21] With the horrors of the 1882 and 1889 epidemics still fresh in many people's minds, there can be no doubt that rumours of the cholera in Manila added to the local elite's demand for an end to guerrilla resistance.

The surrender was supposed to lead to the break-up of the zones of reconcentration, the re-dispersal of peasants in their villages, the preparation of the ricefields, and the reopening of the rice-trade networks. General Bell, having asserted that there was 'absolutely no hunger within the territorial limits of the brigade, and no suffering on that account', admitted that rice was being imported into the region. He was counting on the fact that with the war over 'all land [could] be properly prepared before the planting season'.[22] This was absolutely crucial. The glowing official report on the Tanauan and Santo Tomas 'concentration camps' notes that there was enough rice, including reserves, to last only until 30 April and 1 May, respectively.[23] Search-and-destroy operations by the U.S. Cavalry had destroyed rice stocks which could not be transferred into the zones. Rice aid would enable the people to eat until the September harvest, but the region would only get back on its feet with the normalisation of rice production. Unfortunately, Bell's optimism was soured by complicating factors such as the rinderpest, locusts, and cholera.

The case of Calamba and its adjacent towns illustrates the connection between the food problem and the new round of restrictions occasioned by the cholera. Calamba had been the headquarters of the republican Division of Southern Luzon, commanded by General Juan Cailles. In 1899 there had been fierce battles between U.S. forces and various defence perimeters around Calamba resulting in the destruction of the irrigation works. Thus, no rice had been planted around that town since 1900. When the populace were herded into the town centre in March 1902, work teams were given permission, initially under guard, to repair several dams. It was hoped that rice would be planted that year. In the meantime, the town was rice-dependent on neighbouring Cabuyao and Binan. In February, the American commander of Binan could still inform his Calamba counterpart: 'If it becomes necessary for you to purchase rice for indigent or starving natives, I have a superabundance harvested which the natives are anxious to sell.'[24]

Even before Malvar's surrender, rice had been allowed to enter from neighbouring towns at regular market prices. This, however, was 'suddenly cut off by unexpected quarantine regulations made necessary by the appearance of cholera'. The border between Calamba and rice-rich Binan, in particular, was 'assiduously guarded'. The only rice available was from the U.S. commissary, which was sold to wealthier Filipinos or distributed free to the poor as required. Not surprisingly, frequent attempts were made to run the guard lines. People traversed back lots and rice paddies at night. The situation was aggravated by the fact that May is the month of local feasts honouring patron saints. Apparently, infected food from Manila brought to a feast 'materially assisted' in the infection of Binan.[25]

There are numerous accounts of how quarantine lines disrupted the flow of food from surplus to dependent towns in the provinces of Rizal,

Laguna, and Batangas. There are equally numerous accounts of how, particularly from July, as the rice reserves became depleted in some towns, there was a considerable movement of people seeking to buy or sell rice, fish and other food products.[26] The quarantine was 'absolutely useless', noted Chief Quarantine Officer J. C. Perry, owing to the smuggling of food. He attributed this to 'ignorance' and wished he were dealing with 'intelligent Americans or Europeans instead'.[27] For the inhabitants of the war-torn areas, however, it was ultimately a choice between dying of hunger or dying of cholera. After a period of intense quarantines and house-to-house inspections, the Army had to content itself with isolating or 'protecting' its soldiers from the native populace, or even withdrawing its garrisons.[28]

Even with the ineffectiveness and eventual lifting of the quarantine, the agricultural situation in 1902 was hopeless. Rinderpest, which first appeared on the eve of the 1888 cholera epidemic, had destroyed more than ninety per cent of the work animals. Hand labour, aided in places by hoes provided by the U.S. garrisons, could only work a limited area. The work force was reduced by the ravages of the cholera, not to mention concurrent malarial fever and beriberi.[29] With the cholera sweeping through the region less than a month after the break up of the concentration camps in late April, and with reserve rice running out at the end of that month, southern Tagalog peasants would certainly have been 'debilitated' and 'demoralised'. Only continued rice aid, which Malvar himself petitioned for in August, prevented 'suffering' from turning into a demographic disaster.[30] 'We have cases of cholera in this town', the mayor of San Juan, Batangas, urgently telegraphed Bell in mid-June. 'A lot of people are dying more of starvation than of the cholera, in view of which I beg you to give us protection.'[31]

It may appear that Malvar's surrender and the increasing dependence of the peasants on American food aid effectively ended the war. It can be argued, however, that the war was simply transposed from the battlefields to the towns, that the struggle continued over the control, no longer of territorial sovereignty, but of people's bodies, beliefs and social practices. American military surgeons, the standard bearers of scientific medicine in the colonial world, merely supplanted the officers and combat troops of the initial period of conquest. It was, in a sense, the old war in a new, more complex setting – complex, since who can argue against the saving of human lives through proper disinfection, isolation, treatment, and disposal of the dead?

Sanitary work came in on the heels of General Bell's military offensive beginning in December 1901. As Heiser candidly admits, 'because they had to protect their troops, they decided that something must be done about cholera'. Having made this decision, the Americans were not disposed to tolerate obstacles to health measures.[32] Cholera, in fact, was the lesser problem compared to, as one veteran surgeon wrote, 'an ignorant and suspicious people, impoverished by war, locusts and rinderpest and embittered by conquest', making sanitation work 'an extremely difficult task, calling for much patience, tact and firmness, the brunt of which fell on the Army'.[33]

The rationale for the Army's intervention was to cleanse the regions, to eradicate the dual scourge of killer germ and popular stubbornness. The discourse matches that which framed General Bell's programme for the December military offensive:

> I expect to first *clean out* the Looboo Peninsula. I shall then move command to the vicinity of Lake Taal, and *sweep* the country westward to the ocean and south of Cavite, returning through Lipa. I shall *scour and clean up* the Lipa Mountains. Swinging northward, the country. . . will be *scoured*. . . . Swinging back to the right, the same *treatment* will be given all the country, etc.[34]

Developments in nineteenth-century medicine contributed to the convergence of colonial warfare and disease control. American physicians by 1902 almost universally subscribed to the germ theory, or more generally the doctrine of specific aetiology of disease. Pasteur's writings on the subject appeared at about the same time as Darwin's theory of evolution. At a time when relationships between living beings were being set in a context of a struggle for survival, where one was either friend or foe, the germ theory gave rise to a kind of aggressive warfare against disease-causing microbes, which had to be eliminated from the stricken individual and from the community. When specific pathogenic micro-organisms were discovered after 1870, they were viewed as *the* cause of specific diseases. It was then easy to think of disease as an entity incarnate in the germs and loose in the community. Towards the end of the nineteenth century, medical thinking that recognised the importance of a patient's state of mind, that attributed disease to a lack of harmony between man and his environment, had given way in Europe and America to the search for the specific germ and the specific weapon against it.[35]

Between 1875 and 1900, French and German bacteriologists identified the organisms involved in many of the serious infections like cholera, typhoid and tuberculosis. As is well known, the German doctor Robert Koch discovered the cholera bacillus in the 1880s through investigations conducted in the British colonies of Egypt and

India. Although few cures were to be found until half a century later, implications for preventive measures were apparent. In the United States, sanitary reform proceeded in earnest from the 1870s, spurred on by the public's fears of a recurrence of the cholera visitations of the 1830s and 1850s. By about 1905, control of water or food supplies and of insect vectors had checked typhoid, cholera, yellow fever and malaria.[36]

American surgeons and sanitation personnel, then, had just witnessed the glimmer of victory over disease in their own country when they confronted the cholera in the Philippines. They were armed with the knowledge of Koch's and others' discoveries, of the processes of taming the disease in Europe, America, and the colonies; of its causes, means of prevention, and the treatments available at that time. Their feeling that nothing could hinder them or the march of science is captured by this passage from Inspector General's report of 1902:

> The epidemics among men and beasts have been remarkable since our advent into the Far East. But they come and go like waves, making but little impression upon the national consciousness; for science has seized the recurrent waves and almost obliterated them. Even the bubonic plague has passed, scarce noted. And the struggle goes on. A single sentinel of science remiss may let many suffer.[37]

The tropical environment, the war, and the obdurate populace in particular, were regarded as petty obstacles to the implementation of an unsullied knowledge backed up by science and history. Not surprisingly accounts of operations during the epidemic are suffused with a sense of mission and righteous victory. The following episode is typical: '[In Calatagan, Batangas] most of the natives, being ignorant and superstitious, the latter involving fatalism, had no faith in the efficacy of these measures and were much opposed to the restrictions involved'. Thus, between 21 June and 3 July, 650 died of cholera before the native authorities decided to report the situation to the Americans. Within a week 'the surgeons and soldiers sent there had stopped the ravages of the cholera'.[38]

The cholera war proceeded along familiar military lines. Army surgeons, for one, were armed with trial 'magic bullets' with which to shoot down the bacillus. One widely used drug was benzozone, the ingestion of which was found to burn the mouth and stomach linings. It eventually was diluted and mixed in with solutions used to irrigate the bowels and small intestines. Routine treatments involved the use of benzoyl-acetyl-peroxide, guiacol carbonate, calomel, potassium permangante, two per cent tannic acid, and dilute sulphuric acid. These treatments were really experimental in nature, based on the assumption that some drug ought to be able to attack and destroy the cholera vibrio within the patient. The American doctors' use of such and other, unfamiliar, methods of treatment only brought about an aversion in Filipino cholera patients 'so marked in many instances as to necessitate the use of force in the administering of medicine'.[39] In the end none of the medicine, at least in Heiser's experience in the Philippines, proved of any value.[40]

Of utmost importance in the war was the ability to conduct search and surveillance operations. For this purpose Worcester organised platoons of inspectors led by surgeons from the Army Volunteer brigades. Initially, most of the inspectors were Filipinos. But they were soon relieved owing to their inability to understand that 'these measures, to be effective, must be enforced upon the rich as well as the poor, and the strong as well as the weak'.[41] Americans of all kinds were enlisted: clerks, schoolteachers, policemen and ex-soldiers. Among them were some 'who had slight regard for the natives and who enforced the already distasteful regulation in an unwarranted manner, increasing the popular opposition'. Several of them were killed as a result.[42] In the southwestern Luzon towns, native inspectors and guards continued in service but they were supervised by patrols, often mounted, of white soldiers. Filipino scouts, a ruthless elite force consisting mostly of non-Tagalogs, stood guard over quarantined houses.[43]

The cholera introduced the stern figure of the American army surgeon, less open than the regular military officers to compromise with the local elite. Detailed to most local health boards, army surgeons had little regard for their Filipino colleagues and generally ignored local knowledge gained from previous epidemics. As Captain C. de Mey put it, their job was ideally 'to rule with a rod of steel'. A health officer 'should be the commanding officer of a city when that city is threatened with or has an epidemic, and must be left free to act according to his judgement'.[44] In the context of an epidemic, therefore, the surgeon displaces the military commander. Heiser, though never detailed with the army, speaks for the army surgeon as well in commenting that 'whatever the relative importance of the medical man in other parts of the world, he, and the profesion he represented, *stood first* in the Philippines'.[45]

Various 'combat zones' can be identified in the cholera war. Prominent among them was the issue of confinement. We have seen how quarantine lines crumbled before the more pressing need to obtain or sell food. Quarantine formed part of the broader objective of containing the disease. When the epidemic was first discovered in the Farola district, Worcester's platoons attempted to completely cordon off the area in order to isolate the stricken and whoever had had contact with them. However, 'the disease spread rapidly among the imprisoned people and a continuation of the quarantine would have been inhuman', so the inhabitants were transferred to a detention camp.[46] Several such camps were soon put up in Manila and provincial towns.

Heiser describes how 'uniformed men clattered up with ambulances and without ceremony lifted the sick from their mats and carted them away from their wailing families'. Families could not understand why they were forbidden to follow. 'Four times out of five this was the last they ever saw of their loved ones until shortly they received a curt notice to come to the hospital and claim their dead.'[47] Confinement in hospitals for patients, and in detention camps for contacts, was almost as feared as the cholera itself. For one thing, hospitals during the Spanish regime were regarded as places 'where people so unfortunate as to have no homes to die in might go to end their days. It was almost impossible to get any other class of persons into them'. Thus cholera victims 'sometimes had to be taken to the hospital by force'.[48] Compounding the traditional aversion were some terrifying rumours, current from Manila to Cebu, 'of horrible abuses in the detention camps, and of deliberate murder of patients at the cholera hospitals'. It was said that on arrival, patients were given poisoned vino (a cheap Spanish wine) and instantly dropped dead. There were also tales of strychnine poisoning, occasioned by its necessary use as a heart stimulant.[49]

Strict confinement was premised on the then-prevailing notion in American medicine of disease as a purely biological and physical entity, a foreign agent, which must be excised from the healthy parts of society. The Filipino public, however, largely refused to dissociate the disease from the network of social relationships in which it appeared. Rumours, concealments and evasions were various modes of resistance to an imposed definition of sickness and treatment. The conflict became so intense that a concession had to be made to the 'ignorant classes': tents were pitched on the grounds of cholera hospitals to accommodate relatives or friends of patients. Once or twice daily they were allowed to visit the wards.[50] Filipino doctors were also allowed in to practise their 'mixed treatments' which involved keeping the patient in a familiar and reassuring environment, where his morale as well as body was attended to.[51]

Sometime in mid-May, the removal of contacts to detention camps was finally stopped in Manila since this measure only made concealment of cases the rule. On 1 July, even detention in houses was scrapped. In Batangas and Laguna, General Bell abolished forcible detention on 23 May. Henceforth, people were to be isolated in their houses, over which municipal authorities were to place guards.[52]

During the first few weeks of the epidemic in Manila, not only were members of a stricken household sent off to detention camp, but their house itself was burned down if it happened to be a nipa-palm construction. The cholera germ lay in the filth and vermin associated with infected 'native dwellings', which had to be destroyed, germs and all. Many books on Philippine health and sanitation display that famous photograph of the burning of houses in the Farola district.

The problems with such an efficient means of destroying cholera germs is obvious. An American teacher in Cebu put it this way:

> Many of the poor people see absolutely no way of replacing their houses. It's all very well to tell them that they will be paid the value of the buildings destroyed. They have had too much experience to put much faith in such stories. They would also have to wait six months in order that the usual amount of red tape may be gone through. Where are they to live in the meantime? Better let father or brother die and say nothing about it.[53]

Resistance to burnings took the form of rumours, 'widely circulated', that houses of the poor were burned in order to make room for the 'future dwellings and warehouses of rich Americans'. Because it 'provoked great hostility among the poorer people' house burning was quickly abandoned in Manila in favour of thorough disinfection.[54]

In the provinces, Government Order 66 was implemented which stipulated, among other things, that nipa houses of cholera cases were to be burned, while houses constructed of wood were to be disinfected.[55] The local elite was thus spared. We have only one actual report of a burning in southwestern Luzon – that of a nipa house in a barrio of Calamba valued at $15 (Mexican).[56] But there must have been a lot more. The Philippine Commission government awarded $4624.39 as payment for claims of owners of houses burned down by medical officers in the town of Lumbang.[57] If, say, each of the burned nipa huts at Lumbang cost $15, then up to 308 houses could have been destroyed in that town. This is possible. An American teacher in Cebu could not bring himself to implement the order because 'when a fire once starts in one of these towns, it sweeps over acres and acres before it can be stopped'. He burned only 'one or two crazy old shacks'.[58]

In the towns of southwestern Luzon under General Bell's control, there must have been quite a few medical officers like the one who wrote, 'I went next to Cavite, where cases had occurred in a populous market place. The market was burned down. Result, no more cholera for more than two months.' Before this, Captain de Mey had burned down a house in Malolos, north of Manila.[59] In any case, since the burning of whole barrios outside the zones during General Bell's military offensive had already created mass resentment against the U.S. army, well-meaning measures during the epidemic cannot have been accepted passively. There can be no doubt that the threat of burnings figured largely in the concealment of more than fifty per cent of cholera cases in the region.[60] On 23 May, Bell finally sent out orders that no more houses were to be burned when there were only a few cases involved or where the cholera had already disappeared.[61]

Infected houses were not as much of a problem as the infected cadavers that piled up during a cholera epidemic. In 1882, when Manila experienced an estimated death toll ranging from 13,000 to 34,000, bodies remained unburied for days. San Lazaro district, site of the cholera hospital, was so filled with 'gasses of putrefying flesh' that one could hardly go through it. The government finally intervened with a battalion of engineers to help bury the dead *en masse* in a common pit. The approaches to the Manila cemeteries 'were blocked with vehicles of every description loaded with corpses'.[62]

The same problem arose in 1902. By the end of July, the grounds of Tondo cemetery were filled with cadavers and further burials were banned. As in the past, new cemetery grounds were opened up in the suburbs, but the American government still worried that underground water tables would be infected. Certainly, no mass graves would be dug this time. The government instead preferred a more efficient solution: cremation. But this was not directly imposed. Rather, the Insular board of health decreed that cadavers must be placed in hermetically sealed metallic coffins before being buried in seven-foot deep graves. Otherwise, off to the crematories they would be sent, at government cost.[63] Now how many could afford metal coffins? Again, it was the poor that took the blow.

No Filipino in his right mind approved of cremation. An American teacher, convinced that the 'ideal way' of disposing of bodies was 'to burn them', discovered that 'the very mention of such a thing aroused a storm of superstitious opposition':

> The Filipinos and Spaniards both informed me that it would be a tremendous mistake even to attempt burning any bodies. The natives had such a horror of it that they would rather scoop out a trench under a house in which to bury the dead, or throw the body in the nearest

swamp. I pointed out that in neither case would they be burying their dead in consecrated ground. Even so – that was a good deal better than having the bodies burned.[64]

In Manila hospitals, corpses left unclaimed after twenty-four hours were cremated. In the crowded conditions of the city slums, it was possible during an epidemic's peak for cholera victims to be so regarded with fear and horror as to be abandoned. At least this is what happened in 1888, when victims were 'not infrequently' carried out while in a state of coma and buried alive. Not a few survived and returned to terrorise their friends! It became necessary to issue orders to deposit bodies in shelters and leave them there for a few hours before burial.[65] In 1902, fear of cremation combined with fear of house burnings and fear of detention, forced poorer families to bury bodies in backyards, under woodpiles, or out in the ricefields at night; or even to throw them into the Pasig river.

On 1 July the board of health backed down on its strict burial regulations. 'Owing to the religious prejudices of the people against the cremation', and the consequent concealment of cases, families and friends of persons dying of cholera in Manila could henceforth bury their dead in simple wooden coffins placed in lime-filled graves seven feet deep. On the 29th, the board conceded even more: the graves could be as deep as the condition of the ground permitted, but not less than three feet in any case. However, only two adult members or friends of the family could accompany the body. And no services, funeral processions or bands were to be allowed.[66]

Although the Insular board of health did not recommend cremation for the provinces, this did take place. There were times when the board had to order it to be stopped because none of the provinces had the proper facilities for it. The result of all cremation attempts had been 'to arouse the horror of the people, and their passive, and in some instances active, resistance to such measures and to all general sanitary measures'.[67]

In comparison to Manila's poor districts where overcrowding and intense government surveillance imposed additional pressures and fears on the inhabitants, there were fewer horror stories in provincial towns. The fact that American troops kept to their garrisons in the town centres, was a contributing factor. Army surgeons and their inspectors policed the centre, while in the outlying villages either a vigorous local-led campaign was carried out, or the epidemic was simply allowed to run its course. In neither circumstance could there have been much American interference in the practices surrounding sickness and death.

In the town of Pila, Laguna, for example, the leading citizens were ordered to supervise the digging of about twenty graves daily, ten for grown persons and ten for children. In addition, they had to obtain burial permits from the American commanders and see to it that no excess people accompanied the corpses to the cemetery.[68] But if the people of Pila wished it, the rules could be broken. In the barrios, concealment was a simple matter. Relatives, neighbours and children visited the sick or the dead without constraints. Some came to pay their respects, to join in the feast called *katapusan*; others just wanted to see what the dying and the dead looked like – and cholera victims were a horrible sight. The same utter disregard for prohibitions was reported in towns all over the Philippines. 'They have no fear of anything', sighed a frustrated teacher in the Visayas.[69] At Ibaan, Batangas, infected houses were required to display a red flag, 'but the natives gave no heed to this warning and to them the presence of the flag was seemingly only a kind of joke'.[70] Observers saw this as a sign of fatalism and ignorance. On the other hand, it can be read as an insistence that death and dying remain a social event.

The towns were the scene of conflicts between army surgeons and native officials. Such were the local tensions that Worcester, in touring the provinces, had to discipline some abusive American health officials.[71] Trouble usually erupted when local officials were accused of being incompetent or unco-operative. Provincial and municipal boards of health, composed of Filipinos, were regarded as 'entirely incompetent to meet the emergency of dealing with an epidemic'. In one Laguna town, members of the local health board were imprisoned for 'criminal laxity', that is, not reporting cases to the army surgeon. Uncertainty of diagnosis was the proffered excuse.[72] In the few provinces and towns where success in stamping out the cholera was reported, credit was given to army surgeons on detail with the local boards.

It is hard to accept such charges at face value when we take into account the fact that municipal health commissions, or *juntas sanitarias*, had functioned under similar guidelines during the 1882 and 1888 epidemics.[73] What is missing in American accounts of local bungling or intransigence is precisely the war context or, to put it another way, the local interpretations – shaped by recent memories – of the colonial enterprise of saving human lives from disease.

A brief report from San Pablo, Laguna, states that the army surgeon, Major Isaac Brewer, was engaged in a bitter fight with the mayor over the handling of the epidemic. The mayor was accused of being 'too slow', while Brewer was allegedly 'insulting and impatient'.[74] Was this another one of those ubiquitous cases of native ignorance or stubbornness? In placing this incident in context we discover that just six months earlier the town church had been occupied by U.S. troops and the parish priest detained. The following month, the mayor had been unceremoniously dismissed, presumably for aiding the guerrillas. At the height of reconcentration, the door of the sacristy, where religious objects had been stored under guarantee of safety by the American commanding officer, had been forced open and several gold and silver chalices, ciboriums, albs, and plates stolen. Occupation troops only abandoned the church on around 17 May, the day the parish priest was freed.[75]

We do not know if the parish priest, Father Alcantara, was a party to the local opposition to interference by American health authorities. It is difficult to picture him bowing to an army surgeon after what the troops had done. He could very well have been one of those native priests who were telling people in the confessional that the Americans were making the anti-cholera campaign 'a pretext for harassing them'. This opposition or 'interference' was great enough to provoke the government to warn the highest church authorities.[76] Priests had always taken charge in past epidemics, parading the host around town, leading novenas and processions, dispensing the last sacraments, at times even heading the local sanitation boards. They represented the notion, antithetical to the army surgeons', that sickness was both a moral as well as a physical state.[77]

San Pablo suffered much during the reconcentration and this the townspeople could not be expected to forget so quickly. The town centre was transformed into one of the three largest concentration camps in southwestern Luzon. Yet, when it was found impossible to 'protect' the people scattered along the main roads, the zone was further decreased in size.[78] People were packed even closer together, making a mockery of sanitation and vastly increasing the chances of infection. None were left outside to attend to the ricefields. Even in pre-war years, San Pablo's normal crop was only one-twentieth of demand. Its income from the copra trade enabled nearly all its rice to be bought from neighbouring towns.[79] This revenue was severely cut back by the reconcentration. The copra trade recommenced in late April only to be hampered by the quarantine, the prohibition of lake traffic in June, and other cholera measures. For a while the townspeople survived on rice aid.

Even before the cholera the mortality from dysentery and malarial fever had been enormous in the San Pablo zone, with 362 deaths being reported in March alone. The army surgeon attributed this to the reconcentration, which gave rise to 'crowded conditions and limited facilities' that prevented sanitation and curative measures from being enforced so as to significantly lessen the mortality. He recommended that the natives be permitted to return to their barrios as soon as conditions permitted. If not, 'owing to the generally unhealthy conditions prevailing, an outbreak of cholera would jeopardise the life of every one in the town, both soldier and native'. When the cholera did arrive, the town was still packed with people, now prevented by quarantine from moving out. However, as in several other garrisoned towns, the American troops were able to flee.[80]

Given such circumstances, it is not hard to imagine why the mayor of San Pablo and the American army surgeon were locked in a bitter squabble at the height of the epidemic. We can hardly doubt that Major Brewer was acting in good faith, but his stress on the 'correctness' of his methods ignored the local context. From the townspeople's point of view, the American presence was as much a problem as the cholera. The mayor's irritating 'slowness' was but another form of resistance. Representations of the event as an epic struggle against disease and ignorance only divert attention from the wider, all-encompassing colonial intervention which Filipino participants could not easily forget.

In towns where the overseer of epidemic control was the American garrison commander rather than an army surgeon, the tensions were much reduced. For example at Pila, only some twenty kilometres north of San Pablo, the commanding officer simply instructed the mayor to divide up the town into cholera districts under the headship of prominent citizens many of whom had fought in the resistance. A former guerrilla hero, Colonel Ruperto Relova, was put in charge of two barrios. All dealings with the people such as explaining health measures, reporting cases, and arranging burials, were made through men like him.

Militarily, Pila was of little consequence to the Americans. In July, at the height of the epidemic, the whole garrison was moved out. Furthermore, with a population only a quarter that of San Pablo, and being a traditional rice-surplus area, Pila was able to escape food supply problems. In this case, then, the principales were in control and the U.S. presence was weak. There was no need for a 'poor fund', no dependence on rice aid, no threat of the traditional social order being upset by arrogant army surgeons. No fuss was made about concealment of cases and the like, because none were discovered.[81]

The example of Pila shows how a different tactic by the Americans could lead to mutual accomodation – a truce perhaps – within a combat zone. In fact, it seems to have been the norm that colonial health and sanitation control provoked popular resistance which, in turn, forced concessions to be made such as the elimination of detention, burnings and cremation, and, most crucial of all, the gradual turning over of disease control to Filipino doctors and local authorities.[82] The other side of apparent local victories in such adjustments, compromises, and accomodation of local customs, was that Filipinos were given the space within which to come to terms with colonial state power. In a sense, it was the Spanish conquista all over again.

As the local elites put their towns into line with at least the broader outlines of the colonial sanitation scheme, the government increasingly found itself confronting the traditional 'other' of the Hispanised town-centre. The new colonial order, in fact, merely reproduced the classic Philippine pattern of principalia-dominated, sanitary, towns whose outskirts faded into a world of 'uncontrollable', 'disorderly' or 'subversive' elements. After Malvar's surrender, all forms of armed resistance to the regime were labelled 'ladronism (from the Spanish word *ladron*, 'bandit' or 'highwayman'). A particular form of this which incorporated religious beliefs and rituals was labelled 'religious fanaticism'.

In the Mariquina valley, the Filipino provincial medical officer and his American counterpart appealed at the end of July for an easing of quarantine restrictions for the following reasons: past harvests had been poor; war conditions had hindered planting in the past three years; the previous crop had been destroyed by locusts; now the quarantine was preventing peasants from tilling their fields. Yet tenants were being forced to pay their annual rent, 'crop or no crop'. As a result 'many of them, and many of the field labourers [were] taking to the mountains and joining the ladrones as a means of earning a living'.[83] Were these 'bandits' among those who joined up with the revived Katipunan revolutionary government which began to appear in parts of Cavite, Laguna, Tayabas and Rizal provinces beginning, not surprisingly, in mid-1902?[84]

The foothills of Mount Banahaw, straddling the provinces of Laguna, Tayabas and Batangas, were in a state of unrest in late 1902, to the extent that some Tayabas towns had to be reconcentrated again. Various post-Malvar guerrilla leaders like 'Pope' Ruperto Rios and the Katipunan chief Macario Sakay, roamed these hills in late 1902 and

1903. A 1903 report on the religio-political movements based on these hills states that 'independence' had become a religion among them. 'The magical condition of independencia' was their goal.[85] In Tagalog, the word 'independence' is *kalayaan*, one of whose meanings is derived from *kaginhawaan*: 'relief from pain', 'a life of ease'.[86] 'Relief from the cholera' would certainly have registered in 1902–3. Notably, the 'password' among members of such movements was, and still is, *Ave Maria purissima . . . sin pecada concebida* – the first line of a prayer, posted on doors during the cholera epidemic, imploring the Virgin Mary and Jesus Christ for deliverance from the pestilence.[87]

Banahaw and its foot-hills were the base of operations of *curanderos*, curers who, rather than licensed physicians, were the first recourse of peasants in the region.[88] An American doctor described them as men and women who 'do not constitute a class or caste like the medicine men of savage tribes, but are somewhat akin to the barber surgeons of villages in continental Europe in which doctors are not located'. *Curanderos* commonly prescribed a cholera medicine extracted from the *manungal* tree (*Samadera Indica*) grown in Tayabas province.[89] A particularly gifted curer combined medicinal treatment with rituals involving the intervention of a guiding spirit. A condition of treatment was for the patient to undertake some form of pilgrimage to Mount Banahaw in fulfilment of a *panata*, or pledge, to supernatural beings. Cholera epidemics clearly offered ideal conditions for the appearance of healers who attracted villagers away from town-centres and to their fold.[90]

It was common for colonial authorities in 1902 and subsequent cholera years to forcibly disperse people gathered in places considered to be sources of infection: sacred springs, pilgrimage sites, even churches and cockpits. At times, a proscribed healer was the centre of attention and promptly suppressed; in other cases, the normal ritual life of the people was disrupted. In accounts emanating from garrison commanders, health officers, teachers, and the like, such interventions are justified in the light of problems posed by ignorance and superstition.

But why did such 'problems' persist? As late as 1914, Worcester continued to lament the 'unending supply' of healers such as the 'Queen of Taytay', discovered during another cholera outbreak in 1905, whose hundreds of followers threatened violent confrontation with the state should harm befall their leader.[91] What were the contours of the knowledge that such healers possessed? What lay behind pilgrimages to Antipolo and Banahaw besides 'fanaticism'? The sources are silent.

Little emerges from the world of the native inhabitants that is not mediated, distorted, by the medico-sanitary discourse of the period. Whatever their real nature, such phenomena spelled danger for the representatives – Filipino and American alike – of the new colonial order. Crowds were being dispersed from sources of infection, they argued, but one suspects that such ritual gatherings were equally suppressed for what they forbode of alternative social orderings or sources of disorder.

Cholera cases and deaths in southwestern Luzon declined in September and October. Strong typhoons were lashing the islands then and, as army surgeons themselves noted, the resulting volume of water flushed the streams and banks. The virulence of the 1902 cholera strain had also expended itself by that time; the population gained increasing immunity. In fact, the cholera seemed to follow the course of the great visitation of 1882. But Worcester and other health officials disagreed, attributing the decline of cases to American health and sanitation measures. In terms of preventing further serious outbreaks, such measures, adapted to local conditions, were probably effective. But in 1902 their actual role was to close a chapter of the Philippine–American war.

Notes

An earlier version of this chapter was presented at the conference 'Death, disease and drugs in Southeast Asian history', held at the Australian National University. My thanks to all those who commented on the draft, especially Ben Anderson, Ben Kerkvliet, Norman Owen and Rod Sullivan. A grant from the Ford Foundation Southeast Asian Fellowship Progam enabled me to conduct the U.S. archival work on which this essay is based.

1 T. A. Agoncillo and M. C. Guerrero, *History of the Filipino People*, Quezon City, 1977, pp. 262, 340, 423-5 (on education), 425-6 (on health and welfare).

2 D. C. Worcester, *Asiatic Cholera in the Philippine Islands*, Manila, 1908; D. C. Worcester, *The Philippines Past and Present*, New York, 1914; V. Heiser, *An American Doctor's Odyssey*, New York, 1936.

3 *Asiatic Cholera*, p. 18.

4 'Exemplar of Americanism: the Philippine career of Dean C. Worcester', Ph.D. thesis, James Cook University of North Queensland, 1987, p. 146.

5 Maj. C. Lynch, 'Asiatic Cholera', Circular 24, Headquarters Division of the Philippines, Manila, 11 April 1902, in file 4981-5, United States National Archives, Bureau of Insular Affairs, Record Group 350 (Henceforth cited as U.S.N.A. BIA/file number). An account of the spread of the epidemic to Asia and ultimately the Philippines is found in J. C. Perry, Chief Quarantine Officer, *Public Health Reports*, 17 (henceforth cited as Perry Reports), 26 September 1902, pp. 2240 ff., BIA/4981–9.

6 Annual Report of the Secretary of the Interior to 31 August 1902, in *Reports of the Philippine Commission, 1902*, Washington, 1903, p. 273.

7 Col. L. M. Maus, Commissioner of Public Health, *Report*, 31 July 1902; Appendix A to Worcester, *Annual Report*, pp. 342-3.

8 Chief Surgeon's Report, in 'Annual report of the Third Separate Brigade to 1 July

1902', typescript, file 2354, United States National Archives, Records of U.S. Army Overseas Operations and Commands, Record Group 395 (henceforth cited as U.S.N.A. RG395/file number).

9 Lt. Col. P. Harvey, Chief Surgeon, Div. of North Phil., to Adjutant General, 13 May 1902, U.S.N.A. RG395/2635.

10 Dr S. del los Angeles and Capt. F. W. Dudley, 'Joint recommendations for Mariquina, San Mateo, Montalban', 31 July 1902, U.S.N.A. RG395/E2635–13845.

11 Davis, Adjutant, Third Separate Brigade, to commanding officer, Calamba, 19 April 1902, and to commanding officers of all seaport towns 26 April 1902, U.S.N.A. RG395/3287.

12 Surgeon General's Report, in *Reports of the U.S. War Department*, 1902, House Documents IV, 57th Congress, 2nd session, 1902–3, p. 613; Chief Surgeon's Report, Third Separate Brigade.

13 An American surgeon assured the public that 'the well-to-do in the Philippines, including most of the Americans and Europeans, are protected . . . by the better sanitary conditions under which they live'. They merely had to remain vigilant, particularly against the 'carelessness or ignorance of native or Chinese cooks'; Lynch, p. 8.

14 H. A. Lindley, Report of the Santiago Cholera Hospital, 17 June to 31 July 1902, exhibit F to Maus Report.

15 Chief Surgeon's Report, Division of the North Phil., Manila, 30 June 1902, U.S.N.A. RG395/2635–11535.

16 Pangasinan, north of Manila, is the only other province where the exceptional 'virulence' of the cholera is noted; Surgeon General's Report, 1902, pp. 613-4.

17 Chief Surgeon's Report, Third Separate Brigade. The complex causes of the massive decline in the Batangas population are analysed in G. A. May, '150,000 missing Filipinos: a demographic crisis in Batangas, 1887–1903', *Annales de Démographie Historique*, 1985, pp. 215-43.

18 Dr. F. Bourns, Commissioner of Public Health, Report, August 1902, appendix B to Worcester, *Annual Report*, p. 393.

19 In a recent study of the zones of concentration in Batangas, G. A. May suggests that, in fact, conditions in the camps contributed to the spread of cholera; 'The "zones" of Batangas', *Philippine Studies*, 29, 1981, p. 102.

20 M. Malvar, 'Testimony', Lucena, 16-19 June 1902, U.S.N.A., Records of the Adjutant General's Office, Record Group 94, file 421607 (henceforth cited as U.S.N.A. RG94/file number).

21 Commanding Officer (henceforth C.O.) Calamba to C.O. Santa Cruz, 12 April and 20 April 1902, U.S.N.A. RG395/3284; Post Surgeon, Calamba, to Adjutant, 13 April 1902, U.S.N.A. RG395/3287. Dates of the first appearance of cholera in the provinces, with statistics, to 1 September 1902 are in exhibit A to the Bourns Report.

22 Cited in Maj. Gen. L. Wheaton (Commanding, Div. of North. Phil.), Report, 6 May 1902, in U.S. War Dept., *Annual Reports, 1903*, 9, pp. 232-3.

23 Col. A. L. Wagner, 'Report on the zones of Tanauan and Santo Tomas', 22 March 1902, U.S.N.A. RG395/2635–7788. Wagner admits that the purpose of the report is to combat U.S. public opinion against 'concentration'.

24 C.O. Calamba to Adj. Gen. Third Separate Brigade, 14 March 1902, U.S.N.A. RG395/3284; C.O. Binan to C.O. Calamba, 5 February 1902, U.S.N.A. RG395/3287.

25 Adjutant, Calamba, to Commissary, 1 June 1902, U.S.N.A. RG395/3284; Chief Surgeon's report, Third Separate Brigade.

26 On Rizal, S. de los Angeles to C.O., Mariquina river guard, 19 August 1902, RG395/2635; Harvey to Adj. Gen. Third Separate Brigade. On Laguna: C.O. Pila to Adj. Gen. Third Separate Brigade, 1 March 1902, RG395/4747; C.O. Santo Tomas to Adj. Gen. Third Separate Brigade, 7 August 1902, RG395/2354. On Batangas: C.O. San Jose to Bell, July 1902, RG395/2354; L. Gasser to Adj. Gen. Third Separate Brigade, 1 August 1902, RG395/2354. (all U.S.N.A.)

27 Perry Reports, 2 August 1902.

28 Enlisted men at San Jose (Batangas) were prohibited from leaving the plaza unless

sent on duty, 'not only on account of the cholera but because it prevents any possible friction or unpleasantness between the soldiers and natives'; C.O. San Jose to Bell. The last entry in the Pila record book is 12 July 1902, U.S.N.A. RG395/4747. On the withdrawal from Alaminos (Laguna), C.O. Alaminos to Adjutant at San Pablo, 13 June 1902, U.S.N.A. RG395/5101.

29 Lt. L. Gasser to Adj. Gen. Third Separate Brigade, 28 July and 1 August 1902, U.S.N.A. RG395/2354; W. Freer, *The Philippine Experiences of an American Teacher*, New York, 1906, pp. 140-1.

30 C.O. Santo Tomas to Adj. Gen. Third Separate Brigade, 7 August 1902.

31 Guzman to Bell, 15 June 1902, U.S.N.A. RG395/5058.

32 Heiser, pp. 39, 104. A typical case: the commanding officer of Pila requested large amounts of chemicals from the Chief Surgeon in order to 'disinfect the infected sections of the town and thus save the troops from infection'; C.O. Pila to Chief Surgeon, Division of the Philippines, 24 May 1902, U.S.N.A. RG395/4747.

33 George de Shon, M.D., 'Medical highlights of the Philippine- American war', *Bulletin of the American Historical Collection*, 12, 1984, p. 69.

34 Circular Order no. 22, 25 December 1901, cited in C. B. Elliot, *The Philippines to the End of the Commission Government*, New York, p. 28; my italics.

35 R. Dubos, *Mirage of Health: Utopias, Progress, and Biological Change*, New York, 1959, p. 72; R. H. Shryock, *Medicine in America: Historical Essays*, Baltimore, 1966, pp. 98, 324.

36 Shryock, pp. 23-4, 174-5. The extensive historical literature on the cholera need not be listed here. For a comprehensive study of cholera in the context of nineteenth-century British colonialism, see D. Arnold, 'Cholera and colonialism in British India', *Past and Present*, 113, 1986, pp. 118-51.

37 U.S. War Department Reports, 1902, vol. 1, p. 437.

38 Bell to Adj. Gen., Div. of the Philippines, 2 September 1902, U.S.N.A. RG94/453824.

39 Lindley, pp. 389-90; Lynch, p. 13, 17-18.

40 Heiser, p. 101. In a report from the Santa Mesa cholera hospital Capt. T. Marshall admitted that 'the definite lines of treatment advocated from time to time have never proved of material service in true cholera'; 'Report of Santiago cholera hospital, 27 April to 17 June 1902', exhibit B to Maus Report, p. 363. Lynch (p. 18) mentions the replacement of fluids with normal salt solution through intravenous or interstitial injection – probably the only treatment of real benefit. However, this does not appear to have been widely practised in the treatment of Filipinos, at least in 1902.

41 Worcester, *Annual Report*, pp. 271, 275.

42 J. A. Le Roy, 'The Philippines health problem', *The Outlook*, 71, 13, 26 July 1902, p. 780; Worcester, *The Philippines*, p. 442; Sullivan, pp. 214-15.

43 Chief Surgeon's Report, Third Separate Brigade.

44 C. F. de Mey, 'Cholera Report', 30 May 1902, appended to Worcester, *Annual Report*, pp. 412-13.

45 Heiser, p. 38; my italics.

46 Worcester, *Annual Report*, p. 268.

47 Heiser, p. 106. See also Sullivan, p. 215.

48 Worcester, *The Philippines*, p. 442.

49 Worcester, *The Philippines*, p. 416; Worcester, *Annual Report*, p. 271; Perry Reports, 13 August 1902; Heister, p. 106. Le Roy (p. 781) says that abuses were, indeed, committed but does not give details.

50 Maus Report, p. 344.

51 Lindley, p. 390; Bourns, p. 392. Filipino doctors retained elements of the 'traditional' treatment practised since the 1840s, which is described in J. P. Bantug, *Short History of Medicine in the Philippines during the Spanish Regime, 1565–1898*, Manila, 1952, pp. 36-7.

52 Adjutant, Santa Cruz, to C.O. Pila, 23 May 1902, U.S.N.A. RG395/4748; Maus Report, p. 326.

53 'Teachers and cholera in the Philippines', *The Nation*, 77, 8 October, 15 October 1903.

54 Worcester, *Annual Report*, pp. 269, 271.
55 General Order 66, Headquarters, Div. of the Philippines, 25 March 1902, U.S.N.A. RG395/E3287.
56 C.O. Calamba to Adjutant, 13 April 1902, U.S.N.A. RG395/3287; C.O. Calamba to C.O. Santa Cruz, 20 April 1902, U.S.N.A. RG395/3284.
57 Acts of the Philippine Commission, no. 490, in *Report of the Philippine Commission for 1903*, Washington, 1904, pt. 2, p. 1149.
58 'Teachers and cholera'. At Dagupan, sanitary inspectors set fire to several houses but the fire could not be controlled and the city itself was threatened with destruction; *Manila Times*, 9 July 1902, cited in Sullivan, pp. 209-10.
59 de Mey, p. 412.
60 Fifty per cent is, in fact, a conservative estimate. In the Chief Surgeon's report for the month ending 15 July, he states that 'it is probable that in the whole archipelago not more than one-fourth or one-fifth of the cholera cases are now being reported'; cited in Surgeon General's Report, 1902, pp. 613-14.
61 Bell's instructions mentioned by the Adjutant at Santa Cruz, in a letter to C.O. Pila, 23 May 1902.
62 Bantug, p. 31; Worcester, *The Philippines*, p. 410.
63 Maus Report, pp. 327, 332.
64 'Teachers and cholera'.
65 Worcester, *Annual Report*, p. 269; Worcester, *The Philippines*, p. 410.
66 Maus Report, pp. 326-7.
67 Bourns Report, p. 393. An account of a 'macabre' cremation in Nueva Cáceres, seat of the archbishopric of southern Luzon, is given in Sullivan, p. 210.
68 C.O. Pila to presidente of the town, 4 June 1902, U.S.N.A. RG395/4747.
69 T. Marshall, Chief Health Inspector, 'Asiatic Cholera in the Philippine Islands' (Health Bulletin 2, 1 August 1902), Manila, 1904, U.S.N.A. BIA/4981–20, p. 11; 'Teachers and cholera'; Bantug, p. 36.
70 Report of Capt. L. B. Sandall, cited in Surgeon General's Report, p. 613.
71 Le Roy, p. 781.
72 Perry Report, 2 August 1902; Chief Surgeon's Report, Third Separate Brigade.
73 An American doctor opposed to the imperial take-over pointed out that Americans were simply ignorant of the state of Spanish-Filipino medicine; D. Doherty, 'Medicine and disease in the Philippines', *Journal of the American Medical Association*, 16 June 1900 (reprint), p. 16.
74 Report from post, San Pablo, June 1902, U.S.N.A. RG395/2635–12066.
75 Fr F. Alcantara to Sr Archbishop of Manila, 20 May 1902, U.S.N.A. RG359/2635–12912.
76 Le Roy, p. 781.
77 Freer, p. 146; 'Teachers and cholera'. The crucial role of priests in earlier epidemics is amply documented in the eight *colera* bundles located in the Philippine National Archives.
78 Wheaton Report, p. 233.
79 C.O. Santo Tomas to Adj. Gen., Third Separate Brigade, 7 August 1902.
80 Surgeon, San Pablo Military Hospital, to Post Adjutant, 14 April 1902, U.S.N.A. RG359/5099. This was the situation, as well, in the concentration camps of Batangas province; see May, 'Zones', pp. 99-100.
81 (all U.S.N.A.) C.O. Pila to presidente, 4 June 1902, RG359/4747; C.O. Santa Cruz to C.O. Pila, 13 February 1902, RG359/E4748; C.O. Pila to Adj. Gen., Third Separate Brigade, 1 March 1902.
82 Worcester, *Annual Report*, pp. 271-2; Bourns Report, p. 392; Perry Reports, 31 July 1902.
83 Angeles and Dudley, 'Joint recommendations'.
84 See R. C. Ileto, *Pasyon and Revolution; Popular Movements in the Philippines, 1840–1910*, Quezon City, 1979, chapter 5.
85 Ileto, pp. 229, 233-4; Freer, pp. 136-8.
86 Ileto, pp. 107-8, 234-5.

87 Freer, p. 144. The full text, translated from the Spanish, is: 'Hail Mary, most pure, who conceived without sin,/ Holy God, Holy Strength, Holy Immortal,/ Deliver us, Lord from the pestilence and from all evil./ By thy wounds, by thy cross,/ Deliver us from the pestilence,/ thou divine Jesus.'

88 Hence the saying 'le curo el tonto y le mato el sabio' (the stupid man cures while the learned man kills); Bantug, p. 35. Figures for as late as 1912 show that the towns around the mountain harboured an abnormally high proportion, in relation to trained medical personnel, of curanderos; *Infant Mortality in the Philippine Islands*, Manila, 1914, p. 439.

89 Dohery, p. 16; Fr J. M de Zuniga, *Status of the Philippine Islands in 1800*, orig. pub. 1893, Manila, 1973, p. 417; Bantug, p. 27.

90 From interviews with Dr Consolacion Alaras, University of the Philippines. In 1902, old Visayans who eschewed American medicine reminisced about 'a famous old native medicine-woman from Cebu who wrought miracles with her "santas medicinas" during the 1888 cholera visitation'; 'Teachers and cholera'. On the unrest in Samar occasioned by pilgrimages after the cholera of 1882-3, see B. Cruickshank, *Samar: 1768–1898*, Manila, 1985, chapter 8.

91 Worcester, *The Philippines*, p. 437. Heiser (pp. 122-3) gives a more detailed version of the story.

CHAPTER SEVEN

Plague and the tensions of empire: India 1896–1918

I. J. Catanach

The plague which came to Bombay in 1896 – almost certainly by steamship from Hong Kong – was first diagnosed by an Indian practitioner of western medicine, a Dr Viegas. (Most of the official documents insist on calling him 'Mr Viegas'.) Plague had hardly been known in India for several centuries. Only grudgingly was it admitted by the British authorities, in late September 1896, that there were a few cases of 'bubonic fever' of a 'mild' type.[1]

Even then, some scepticism remained in European circles. After all, the original diagnosis had been made by one of those 'qualified (or otherwise) local practitioners'[2] who had recently begun to make their presence felt not only in medicine but also in Bombay political circles.[3] Viegas insisted on trumpeting his discovery before the Standing Committee of the Bombay Municipal Corporation, of which he was a member. R. H. Vincent, the city's Police Commissioner told the Standing Committee not to jump to conclusions about this 'fun'.[4] Vincent had public order considerations in mind; colonial rule, it has been pointed out often enough, depended on 'collaboration', of a sort, from many sections of the ruled. Other Europeans had economic considerations – at least to some extent shared by the important Indian industrialist element in Bombay. The *Bombay Gazette*, a non-official newspaper, cautioned against 'exaggerated statements which might be injurious to the trade and industries by which the city prospers'.[5] Confirmation of the existence of plague came on 12 October 1896 from the bacteriologist W. M. Haffkine – of whom we shall hear more. But on the same day the *Bombay Gazette* was 'glad to report that the sickness is rapidly being stamped out'.[6] Soon, three million gallons of carbolic acid and salt water were being pumped daily through Bombay's drains and sewers: surely all would be well in a short time.[7]

The very facts of the colonial situtation probably demanded that there be such a display of confidence at this stage. Western medicine, or at least a belief in the efficacy of western medicine, helped to make life tolerable for Europeans in India – and, as the *Times of India*, another Bombay newspaper, told its readers in 1898: 'Englishmen believe that England has shown the way to the rest of the world in sanitary science.'[8] Western medicine helped to give what has been called the 'illusion of permanence' to British rule in India.[9] It was, to use the words of Daniel Headrick, one of the 'tools of empire'.[10]

Yet in India, in reality, western medicine shared in the insecurities and the tensions within imperialism. Just as the coming of plague highlighted political, communal and class differences within Indian society[11] – very much as other epidemic diseases have done in other places and other societies[12] – so, too, amongst the rulers of India, the coming of plague for a time exposed the 'illusion of permanence' for what it was. Rivalries and differences between the British government and the Government of India, between various provincial governments, between the various imperial services, between officials and non-officials, and, above all, between individuals – all were, for a comparatively brief moment, rather starkly revealed.

In 1896, for all the activity and all the appearance of omniscience, little of any consequence was known by European medicine, in India or elsewhere, about the aetiology of plague. Next to nothing was known about its treatment. Western medicine had yet to discover the vital role (at least in this, the most recent pandemic) of the flea: the flea which bites humans after deserting a plague-infested rat or other rodent. Early in 1897 a number of Bombay's leading allopathic practitioners, European and Indian, were brought to endorse a statement drawn up by Surgeon-General James Cleghorn, Director-General of the Indian Medical Service (I.M.S.), which asserted that plague was 'only slightly contagious or infectious', and that its incidence was 'greatly due to local conditions'.[13] Cleghorn's opinions were, as it happened, not entirely incorrect, but some of his backers tended to hold old 'miasmatic' views. (After all, as late as 1894 the troops of the Indian Army were supposed to march at right angles to the wind when cholera was about.)[14] It was only in May 1899, after Cleghorn had retired, that he was brought to admit his basic ignorance about plague.[15]

Most of the members of the I.M.S. – certainly those of Cleghorn's generation – saw the Service as an alternative to general practice, of a frequently unprofitable variety, in Great Britain. They were not uninterested in new developments in medicine, but, like most general practitioners, they were not especially research-minded. By the later 1890s the situation was beginning to change, but it is significant that even in 1899 Ronald Ross felt obliged to leave the Service because of inadequate support for his malaria research. Some members of the I.M.S. spent all their working careers in the service of the Indian Army. In a formal sense, indeed, all members of the I.M.S. remained, during the whole of their time in India, army officers, liable to be recalled to military employ. But the aim of many was a Civil Surgeoncy in a large district town. Here they could combine official work with private practice – although many were now experiencing some competition from 'local practitioners', graduates of the Indian medical colleges. Work in the 'sanitary', or public health, sphere was unpopular, partly because it did not allow much private practice.[16]

To some extent the I.M.S. experienced the closing of the ranks against all things Indian which seems to have marked the Indian services in the later nineteenth century. It experienced, too, the 'professionalising' activities of practitioners of allopathic medicine throughout the English-speaking world at this time.[17] In the key province of the Punjab the links between official medicine and Indian medicine, that of the *hakims* and the *vaids*, were virtually severed in 1889.[18] Yet Cleghorn, while serving in the Punjab, had sought more openings for Indians as Civil Assistant Surgeons;[19] his successor as Director-General of the I.M.S., Robert Harvey, was possibly of an even more liberal inclination in matters of race.[20] The I.M.S. never completely shut its doors to non-Europeans. In this way – but more emphatically in other ways – the I.M.S. rather self-consciously differentiated itself from the Army Medical Service (soon to become the Royal Army Medical Corps), which had representatives serving with British regiments temporarily stationed in India. The I.M.S. also felt rather superior to the Colonial Medical Service, which operated in the crown colonies. For all that, however, the I.M.S. was, at the time of plague's coming to India, the poor relation, in terms of financial reward and in terms of prestige, of the Indian Civil Service. To some extent it shared in that subordination of military power to civil power that Curzon sought to reinforce in his confrontation with Kitchener in the early years of the twentieth century.

At the end of 1896 and early in 1897 the Bombay plague mortality figures quite suddenly began to rise. The panic exodus from the city that the authorities had wanted to guard against occurred. Plague broke out in Poona and in the Bombay hinterland more generally. Other European powers began to show signs of agitation: the special fears that the word 'plague' has inspired in the West since the Black Death should never be forgotten. There was talk of the closing of ports to passengers and cargo from India,[21] and even, it was said by the French, a possibility of riots in Marseilles,[22] which had considerable contact with the East and folk memories of an outbreak of plague as late as the 1720s.[23] Bombay soon saw an influx of 'foreign' investigative missions,[24] and the European powers, especially the colonial powers, insisted on calling an International Sanitary Conference in Venice. (There was ample precedent for such a conference.)[25] The reaction of the Government of India to all this was not to doubt the efficacy of western medicine as such. But there were the first signs of doubt about its actual practitioners in India. Cleghorn was despatched to the Venice Conference; he was told, however, that he should stick closely to the British delegate, and that it would be 'not advisable to urge upon the conference any argument founded on the opinion that the plague is not communicated by infection or contagion'.[26] At the conference the French, sometimes adopting a devastatingly 'ironical' tone,[27] took every opportunity to belabour the British, rulers of the home of cholera, and now rulers of one of the epicentres of plague. In the end the British largely got their way: quarantine of passengers and goods coming from India was to be a rarity. But the lesson of such events as the Venice Conference was not lost on the British, either at 'home' or in India: the outbreak of plague had, amongst other things, provided other colonial powers with a pawn in the imperial game. What followed – sometimes awesome regulations, apparently vigorous enforcement of those regulations, and the publication of lavishly produced reports and collections of documents on the plague in India[28] – was to quite a considerable extent the result of an awareness of this fact.

Yet we must beware of being taken in by the published reports, by the contemporary governmental public relations machines. Plague did lead to a rather more vigorous governmental response in India than, say, cholera or smallpox had provoked earlier in the century.[29] The state in India in the last years of the nineteenth century was generally in a more interventionist mood that it had been,[30] and somewhat less inclined to take account of Indian ways and Indian fears. 'The Government has grown harder and more interfering of late years', the young Harcourt Butler wrote to his sister in April 1897.[31] But, when it came to the actual mechanics of plague management at that time, the state in India, with its many concerns, was still often remarkably powerless. 'When you have famine, plague, and a frontier war all on at once, you must be disorganized', B. B. Grayfoot, the secretary to the Bombay Surgeon-General, referring to the situation in his department in the early days of plague, told the Indian Plague Commission.[32]

To this situation there came, at the behest of the India Office, a representative of another facet of empire, Dr James A. Lowson, of the Colonial Medical Service. Lowson had been in Hong Kong at the time of its outbreak of plague in 1894. The authorities in Hong Kong in 1894 had used the army, and even the gunboat, to enforce the hospitalisation of the sick, and so-called 'segregation' of contacts.[33] Lowson believed that similar tactics were required in India. 'It must always be remembered', he pronounced, 'that the plague bacillus is not influenced by diplomacy.'[34] Lowson's own lack of diplomacy increasingly roused India's rulers as he progressed through India: 'anything more impertinent (I can use no other word) I never saw', wrote Lord Elgin, the Viceroy, to the Secretary of State for India.[35] But Lord Sandhurst, the Governor of Bombay, took to heart much, though not all, that Lowson said. The city of Bombay was given over to an army general. In Poona, Walter Rand, the Indian Civil Service officer who was placed in charge of plague matters there, listened hard to another doctor with Hong Kong experience, W. W. Beveridge of the Army Medical Service.[36] Vigorous digging up of earthen floors (where Beveridge believed the plague bacillus resided), thorough disinfecting operations, and above all frequent house-to-house searches for plague victims by British soldiers, followed. The delegation of German doctors sent to India to investigate the epidemic were reported to be 'highly pleased' with what they observed in Poona.[37]

Towards the end of June 1897 Walter Rand was assassinated.[38] In its way, Poona had shown that, unlike Hong Kong, it was not a passive, politically unsophisticated part of the Empire. The Rand murder, coming as it did at roughly the same time as a military defeat on the North-West Frontier, and the first anti-European riot in Calcutta's nineteenth-century history, temporarily caused some Englishmen in India to ask whether 1857 was about to be repeated.[39] Behind the 'illusion of permanence' lay, in fact, considerable insecurity, insecurity that can be summed up in the phrase 'mutiny-watching'.[40] The insecurity of officialdom in India is reflected in the fact that, in the reconsideration of events leading up to the Rand murder that inevitably followed, it became commonplace in official and quasi-official circles to blame Beveridge and Lowson, the 'Hong Kong doctors', rather than Rand, for any 'excesses' that might have occurred in Poona.[41] The Indian Civil Service, to which Rand had belonged, could thus keep its reputation intact, and the Indian Medical Service could take vengeance on its rivals, the Army Medical Service and the Colonial Medical Service.

Nevertheless Surgeon-Major W. L. Reade, of the Army Medical Service, another 'Hong Kong doctor', was in charge of plague operations in Poona from late 1897 until February 1900. He was reported to draw more in pay, with allowances, than the Bombay Surgeon-General himself.[42] He was not above carrying on a self-glorifying correspondence with Arthur Godley, the permanent head of the India Office. 'I consider', wrote Reade, 'that plague operations properly undertaken present some of the best opportunities for riveting our rule in India', and 'also for showing the superiority of our Western science & thoroughness.'[43]

But the reality was that, in spite of 'Western science and thoroughness', plague kept on returning, and spreading. It was above all this fact which gave importance to the activities of one who came to be seen as a dangerous challenge to the medical primacy of the I.M.S., in the Bombay Presidency and beyond. This was a person we have already mentioned, Waldemar Haffkine.[44]

Haffkine had been born a Russian Jew. A conspiratorial student life had been followed by self-exile in Paris. There he was associated with the ageing Pasteur, amongst others. In 1892 Haffkine developed a technique of inoculation against cholera.[45] He was permitted to test it in India, but, partly because of his Russian origins, his activities near the North-West Frontier were a cause of some suspicion at a time when British fears of Russia were considerable.[46] As soon as Haffkine heard of the outbreak of plague in Bombay he offered his services to the Government of India. The authorities swallowed their doubts on the political front, enrolled him in their service, and sent him off to the plague-smitten city. He was certainly the most experienced bacteriologist in the country – one of the very few people with any bacteriological training, in fact – but he brought with him to Bombay a reputation about which there had already been some dispute.

By December 1896 Haffkine, in an ill-equipped laboratory, had developed with he called a plague prophylactic. Early in the new year he had himself secretly inoculated with his new vaccine. He then had it tested on some prisoners – volunteers – in a local gaol. They survived the epidemic much better than those who had chosen not to be inoculated. There, however, the matter could well have rested, at least for some time – had it not been for the fact that plague returned to Bombay, and its hinterland, in 1897–8. In these circumstances there were those – and they included some of Bombay's politically-conscious allopathic doctors – who began, with some encouragement from Haffkine, to talk of large-scale inoculation as an alternative to the more vigorous measures then in vogue.[47]

Surgeon-General G. Bainbridge, head of the I.M.S. in Bombay, would have nothing to do with inoculation. The 'efficiency' of the prophylactic, he wrote, was 'not yet proved'. And he asserted that the broth in which the plague vaccine was cultivated was derived from the flesh of either cows or pigs.[48] Again let us note how 1857 – and its greased cartridges – had not been forgotten. Bainbridge did not voice his concerns only to officialdom; he broadcast them also to the local (European-dominated) Chamber of Commerce. 'Even the "odium theologicum" pales before the jealousy of doctors', commented the Viceroy when he heard of this last incident.[49]

In a sense Haffkine had offended the I.M.S. 'establishment' in Bombay simply by being there. He had bacteriology; they had not. They were doctors; he was not a doctor. Pasteur had had similar problems. But there was more to the matter than this. Haffkine's ideas were being taken up by a section of Indian society that was perceived by many of the I.M.S. as something of a professional, and a political, threat: the 'local practitioners'. And in a sense Haffkine offended in that he was a slightly aloof, hard-working foreigner, and a Russian Jew at that.

One person who had befriended Haffkine before he went to Bombay[50] was another 'outsider' of a sort, William Simpson, Calcutta's city Health Officer.[51] Simpson was not a member of the I.M.S. but was employed by the politically volatile Calcutta Corporation. He was not, in a formal sense, anyway, responsible to the government authorities.[52]

As early as October 1896 Simpson claimed to have discovered a number of cases of plague in Calcutta. The reaction of the Government of Bengal was impressive. It swiftly empanelled a 'Medical Board', heavily weighted with I.C.S. and I.M.S. officers. This Board pronounced that the supposed plague cases were not plague at all, but a type of venereal disease.[53] Calcutta business, especially that part of it concerned with tea and jute export, breathed a great sigh of relief. At the same time, however, at the height of the scare, many Calcutta Europeans – chiefly non-official – worked themselves into a frenzy about the 'insanitary' state of the city. As a result, the first moves were taken that led to the severe abridgement of the Calcutta Corporation's powers in the Calcutta Municipal Act of 1899. Plague provided an appropriate occasion for an assault on what had been, for some years, to a considerable extent the preserve of talkative but supposedly dilatory Bengali *babus*.[54]

It is just possible that Simpson was wrong in his diagnosis of plague in 1896. But Simpson was no fool; he went on to make a distinguished career in epidemiology after he had been virtually forced out of his post in Calcutta. Before he left Calcutta, Simpson compounded his error in the eyes of officialdom by sticking, publicly, to his diagnosis. 'His obstinacy and conceit are beyond control', exclaimed Herbert Risley, Secretary of the Municipal Department of the Government of Bengal.[55] When plague – undoubted plague – broke out in Calcutta in 1898 the Government of Bengal took all control of plague matters out of the hands of Nield Cook, Simpson's successor as Health Officer – who had in any case offended by suggesting that all the disinfection in Bombay did not appear to have done much good.[56] It is significant that in Bengal, too, at this stage, plague control did not go to the I.M.S. It went basically to Risley, the Secretary of the Government of Bengal's Municipal Department. Plague was seen as too important a matter to be left in the hands of doctors.

In a sense this was even more true when plague began to spread out into the rural areas of the Punjab, and to threaten the towns of northern India. It was feared that if plague sprang up in the towns of the north, popular feeling would make it impossible to implement so-called 'segregation' of contacts to the extent that regulations of February 1898 had laid down. Again, in the minds of India's rulers – and this was particularly the case with Sir Antony MacDonnell, Lieutenant-Governor of the North-West Provinces – 'political' considerations ultimately had to take precedence over medical considerations.[57] Again let us note the need of imperialism for tacit 'collaboration': India's British rulers were not operating on a *tabula rasa*.

There was a further, more ruthless, side to changing attitudes to plague administration amongst some of India's rulers. A letter to the editor of the *Civil and Military Gazette* of Lahore put it this way:

> Why on earth should we go on spending crores of rupees on a thankless task . . . Let the natives have the attendance and advice of their professional 'hakims' and be happy and contented, and when the plague has killed half the population of India and spent itself, then perhaps, the native will percieve [sic] the force of the saying. Quos Deus vult perdere, prius dementat.[58] [Those whom God has a mind to destroy, He first deprives of their senses.]

This groundswell of opinion, opposed – for various reasons – to a stringent implementation of plague regulations, was one to which Robert Harvey, who became head of the I.M.S. early in 1898, was able to attach himself. His 'Note on Plague Administration', dated 18 April 1898, was not an entirely independent initiative:[59] given the real position of the I.M.S. *vis à vis* the I.C.S., it could not be. Still, that Note was important. In it Harvey wrote: 'We have to face facts, and the history of the different outbreaks seem[s] to indicate that when once the disease has obtained a firm footing it cannot be stamped out, and . . . attempts to do so by compulsory interference with the habits and the customs of the people do not succeed.' Harvey did hold out some hope, however: he pointed out, very acutely, that the plague visitation in Bombay 'has been a mere trifle compared to very many others of which we have particulars'. Only a little over three per cent of Bombay's population had perished so far. While we now know that at least another ten million Indians were to die from plague over the next twenty years, we also know that except in a very few cases the third plague pandemic was not going to prove to be, in India and elsewhere, nearly so disastrous demographically as the second pandemic, that which struck Europe in 1348. In that pandemic pneumonic cases were probably far more common.[60]

Harvey's memorandum led to a great deal of discussion at a high level, a conference of plague administrators in Simla, the almost inevitable strong dissension from Bombay, and eventually a Government of India resolution which said that the Government was 'not . . . prepared to accept Dr Harvey's conclusions as to the extent to which plague measures hitherto in force have been effective in checking plague'.[61] In other words, the Indian Government was not admitting that it had been wrong. But a good deal of *de facto* relaxation of plague regulations in northern India followed – indeed misunderstandings over differences between formal regulations and their interpretation in practice appear to have been one of the factors behind a serious riot in Cawnpore in 1900.[62] The severe regulations now remained in being mainly to satisfy the 'less enlightened' European powers, as one official called them.[63] Meanwhile, in a rather important *volte face*, it was laid down that practitioners of Indian medicine, *hakims* and *vaids*, could be employed for the supervision of 'public and private hospitals and camps'.[64] In the Punjab, in the years that followed, *hakims* and *vaids* still in fact felt that official policy was stacked against them, and at times still worked against official plague policy. Nevertheless a tentative new beginning in the recognition of indigenous medicine had been made, if still only out of necessity, even despair, rather than out of conviction.

There was one further – and major – consequence of the Harvey memorandum. J. P. Hewett, the Secretary of the Government of India's Home Department, saw the Viceroy and persuaded him to agree, after some initial hesitation, to ask the home government to appoint a commission which would inquire particularly into the 'scientific' aspects of plague, and especially into 'the effects of the preventive inoculation of M. Haffkine'.[65] The India Office agreed – to what was basically, it must be noted, an I.C.S. initiative.

The papers connected with the selection of the membership of the Indian Plague Commission provide an interesting sidelight on the preoccupations of the India Office in respect of plague. The elderly Lord

Lister was consulted, as he so often was in such matters. He recommended as members, amongst others, two of the *bêtes noirs* of many in India: Haffkine (preferably as president of the Commission), and Professor William Simpson, lately of Calcutta.[66] Godley at the India Office promptly replied that, for 'political' reasons, the members of the Commission would have to be people with no experience of the present epidemic – but he then went on to appoint as members of the Commission two Indian Civil Servants who had been closely connected with plague administration.[67] One of them was none other than J. P. Hewett, a man obviously on the way up. The Plague Commission's secretary, furthermore, was a Civilian. The I.M.S., to its disgust, gained no representation on the Commission.[68] Instead, places went to an F.R.S. from Edinburgh;[69] a senior officer in the quasi-imperial medical administration in Egypt (which was known to oppose Haffkine's plague inoculations);[70] and Professor Almroth Wright, of the Netley training establishment for entrants to the I.M.S. and the Royal Army Medical Corps. Wright was a comparatively young man, and had a distinguished career as a bacteriologist in front of him. He was already beginning to gather about himself a small group of disciples in the bacteriological area amongst the I.M.S. trainees.[71]

Yet in spite of Wright's presence the Plague Commission achieved little in the scientific field. Its report was only lukewarm about Haffkine's vaccine,[72] although it put less faith in the rival serum offered by the Frenchman Yersin.[73] The Commission was still more sceptical about another product of French science, the rat–flea theory of the causation of plague. This had been put forward by Paul-Louis Simond (in what is now regarded as a classic paper),[74] only about a month before the Commission began its deliberations. At least the Commission noted the appearance of this paper, and consulted G. H. F. Nuttall, the distinguished parasitologist, and the Hon. Charles Rothschild, the first – but not the last – in that many-faceted family to have an abiding interest in fleas. Simond relied more on induction than experiment: this was the Commission's great objection to his theory.[75] It was a genuine enough objection, although there is some evidence that Simond, from the time in 1897 when he was left to work alone in a couple of tents in Bombay, felt that British India was against him and his country.[76] What the Commission failed to consider was the fact that real scientific 'breakthroughs' are often made as a result of flashes of intuition – leaps beyond the Kuhnian 'paradigms'[77] – rather than as a result of long experiment.

All in all Harvey was right in asserting that the report of the Plague

Commission basically endorsed the policy towards plague which had been followed since he had taken over the I.M.S.[78] But he probably had to thank the I.C.S. members of the Commission for that – and the policy of 1898 and the following years was in any case basically an I.C.S. policy. The Plague Commission report was, at least to some extent, yet another public relations exercise. It is significant that Wright, although he was and still is thought to have been the author of at least some sections of the report,[79] was soon moving, in his possibly slightly devious way, well beyond the conclusions of the report, both in his own work and in the work he encouraged in others.[80]

For all its apparent domination by the I.C.S., however, the Plague Commission did make a plea for an increased emphasis on the 'sanitary' side of the activities of the I.M.S., and, within that emphasis, the development of more research on tropical diseases in India, at a Central Research Institute and in the provinces.[81] This was a potentially important move: the scientists were apparently to be given a greater role. Although the report did not say so directly, by this stage a few of Wright's young protégés were ready and willing to take up the challenge thus offered.

Meanwhile, in 1901–2, the rural districts of the Punjab suffered severely from plague. Not everyone was greatly alarmed by this fact. A correspondent of the *Pioneer*, a newspaper much read by officialdom in northern India, wrote in March 1902: 'We Europeans are indifferent, for the statistics show that fewer Europeans have died from plague than die each year from cholera, so we can chance plague as we chance cholera.'[82] The basic feeling of insecurity amongst Europeans in India which plague had brought out into the open was now beginning to be disguised again behind bluster and cynicism.

But Sir Charles Rivaz, Lieutenant-Governor of the Punjab, was, like most officials in India, looking for a 'success' with which his name could be permanently associated. That would seem to be one reason why, in spite of the hesitancies of the Plague Commission only a little over a year before, he decided upon a campaign of mass inoculation in his province.[83] The Government of India gave him money, and Haffkine was in effect asked to turn his laboratory into a factory, where his prophylactic would be mass-produced. He consented – against his better judgement, one would like to think, but Haffkine, whatever his other virtues, had a strong streak of vanity, and he, too, had a desire for 'success'.

In all, almost half a million Punjab villagers were inoculated with

Haffkine's vaccine in the season 1902–3.[84] This in itself was a considerable bureaucratic and medical achievement, especially in the Indian context. Yet it was an achievement of some fragility. For one thing, it was an 'open secret that inoculation measures in the Punjab were far from being entirely voluntary'.[85] There were rumours that the 'plague doctors' were really 'poisoners'. Then, on 30 October 1902, at a village called Malkowal, nineteen of those inoculated contracted tetanus and died. It is true that Rivaz's scheme did not immediately come to an inglorious end; for a time some inoculations continued to take place.[86] But there was no doubt that the incident was highly embarrassing, not only to the Government of the Punjab but also to the Government of India. It appears very likely that a consignment of the prophylactic became contaminated when an Indian assistant dropped on the ground some forceps used to open the bottle.[87] But the operating doctor, a Dr Elliot, also ought to bear some of the responsibility. He was one of a batch of thirty-seven British doctors temporarily recruited for the inoculation campaign; he was not a member of the I.M.S. One of these doctors was so hopeless that he had to be sent home as soon as he set foot in the Punjab; three others soon followed.[88] As for Dr Elliot, a colleague was brought to comment that he 'always understood that his strong point was romance'.[89]

The full story of the events at Malkowal took some time to emerge. Even Haffkine himself at first thought that the mishap was probably the result of contamination at his laboratory in Bombay.[90] This was at least a possibility, as the Government of Bombay had been very tardy in supplying him with the soldiers he had requested in an effort to fulfil the demands of the Government of the Punjab. The prophylactic was in fact being made by people not inaccurately described at the time as 'half literate boys and newly engaged coolies'.[91]

The Government of India attempted to pin the whole blame for the inoculation fiasco on Haffkine. He had, they said, changed the process of manufacture without informing the Government of Punjab. The documents in the National Archives of India show a quite staggering determination on the part of many, from Curzon, the Viceroy, downwards, to crush Haffkine.[92] The Director-General of the I.M.S. at the time – one who bore the illustrious name of Benjamin Franklin – was on the whole a willing party to the campaign against Haffkine. But for much of the time the lead was taken by Herbert Risley, that ruthless administrator – seen by John Morley as 'somewhat mephistopholean'[93] – now translated from Bengal to the secretaryship of the Home Department of the Government of India. Haffkine, Risley wrote, 'is exceedingly clever; he has means of his own and is I believe about to marry a rich Jewess in Bombay – he will make a remarkably good fight for his reputation'.[94] In fact Haffkine never married, but he did make a good fight.

The Government of India brought in Sir Lawrence Jenkins, who was gaining a reputation as 'the best judge in India',[95] and induced him to change, on a technicality, his commission's initial report on the incident, which did not always show the administrators in the best of lights.[96] Primarily as a result of the Jenkins Commission's Report Haffkine found himself basically 'on leave', for over three years, from his post as Director of the Bombay Bacteriological Laboratory. During some of this period he was unpaid. Haffkine used this time, however, to muster support, in England and in Europe. Those who were induced to come to his assistance included Ronald Ross – hard done by, it will be remembered, in his I.M.S. days – and William Simpson, formerly of Calcutta. A long and carefully argued letter, signed by Ross and Simpson, amongst others, was eventually published in *The Times*.[97] The result – though even then it was not the immediate result – was that Haffkine was re-employed by the Government of India. But he was not given back his old job in Bombay. Nor was he given, as had been promised before the Malkowal affair, the position of Director of the Central Research Institute which had been proposed by the Plague Commission, although he was given the salary he had been promised earlier. He spent most of his remaining time in India, until his retirement in 1915, brooding in a a small laboratory in Calcutta, increasingly bound up in himself and in Judaism. He made little further contribution to the struggle against plague.

The mood of many civil officials at this time, so far as plague was concerned, may perhaps be summed up by Harcourt Butler, rapidly making his way in United Provinces governing circles: 'Our experts perpetually mislead us; and until we have got rid of them we shall have no peace.'[98] There was not much hope for the I.M.S. in these circumstances. Butler was inclined to endorse the 'policy' towards plague of a number of district officers in his province: that of 'do-nothing'.[99]

In his Budget speech of 1907, when plague was at its height in the Punjab, the Viceroy of the time, Lord Minto, asked why so little was said about 'the perennial harvest of the plague'. His private secretary, J. R. Dunlop Smith, felt obliged to explain this 'apathy'. He wrote to Minto:

> The history of the efforts made by Government to combat the plague is a melancholy one. These have lasted for over ten years and have produced practically no results . . . No remedy for plague has been discovered, and inoculation, the only prophylactic found to be of any use has been thoroughly discredited. Evacuation [from the scene of an outbreak of plague] is neither a remedy nor a prophylactic, but it has proved to be a most effective palliation, effective, however, only so long as it lasts. Of late, rat-killing has been resorted to as freely as the resources of Government and the prejudices of the people permitted, but it is too early to say whether this particular plan of operations will meet with any more success than the others . . . Hitherto with our accustomed energy and self-confidence we have been trying to do everything for the people, and we have only succeeded in rousing their prejudices and irritating their religious and social susceptibilities.[100]

This was, in many ways, a succinct summing up of official policy towards plague over the past decade. Once it had been seen that the epidemic was not going to be of the proportions of 1348, once the fears of Europe had to a large extent been allayed, the attitude of many officials in India had, as Dunlop Smith said, lapsed into something approaching 'apathy'. That word, like the word 'fatalism', had long been applied, not altogether fairly, to the attitude of many Indians towards plague – certainly to their attitude after the initial outbreaks.[101] Arguably, the British, for all their 'accustomed energy and self-confidence' (to use Dunlop Smith's words) had now reached a position that was little different from that of many of their subjects.

Dunlop Smith did mention, however, one new development: 'rat-killing'. Prizes were now being offered for numbers of rat-tails being brought into dispensaries and the like. This policy had no great success in the years to come: for one thing, caste Hindus could have little to do with such activities. It needs to be asked, however, why, in 1907, there was this new interest in rats in connection with plague. The reason was that, at last, Simond's rat-flea theory was beginning to find some acceptance in India.

In the world at large, and especially in the Australasian world, the work of Ashburton Thompson and Frank Tidswell of Sydney, and of the brilliant if eccentric J. S. C. Elkington, is seen as providing much of the confirmation that Simond's work required.[102] This view is correct in its essentials; these Australian studies on plague mark the somewhat unexpected, but soon very fruitful, entry of another part of the British Empire into the field of tropical medicine.[103] More than most Indian cities, Sydney – which suffered minor plague epidemics in 1900 and 1902 – was blessed with a stable bureaucracy, and a stable population base for statistical analysis.

However, it must be made clear that Ashburton Thompson was not unaware of the work that was going on in India. Elkington himself visited Bombay at a critical time in 1903.[104] Indeed it appears to have been Elkington who, perhaps a little unfairly, announced to the scientific world beyond India the early discoveries of a young Scots member of the I.M.S., Glen Liston.[105]

In India it was Liston who did most to give the rat-flea theory respectability.[106] He was one of the protégés of Wright who had assisted the Plague Commission in its inquiries. Wright encouraged Liston to persist in his work on the rat-flea, in spite of the published conclusions of the Commission, and in spite of considerable opposition from Haffkine, in whose laboratory Liston now worked. Haffkine quoted the Plague Commission's view on Simond against Liston. In any case, he said, *he* was the scientific head of his laboratory, and those under him should be engaged on *his* work. In March 1903 he gave orders for the dismantling of Liston's apparatus.[107] Such an attitude derived in part from the tension induced in Haffkine by the Malkowal affair, and in part from the Continental laboratories in which Haffkine had worked. It was not derived from peculiarly Indian or even peculiarly British practice. Nevertheless, an antipodean might suggest that it was an attitude that would not have been frequently found at the turn of the century in the small New South Wales Board of Health.

As it happened, it was from a sojourn in New South Wales that, in 1903, the Lister Institute for Preventive Medicine in London drew a new Director, Charles Martin.[108] In September 1904, the India Office approached the Lister Institute for advice on the control of plague. The Institute suggested that control could be more easily accomplished if more were known about the causes of the disease.[109] So there came into being the Advisory Committee for the Investigation of Plague in India. Martin travelled to India, and during some months there recruited Liston and, soon, George Lamb, another I.M.S. officer with bacteriological training, to undertake detailed research work in India. Liston was specifically singled out for this work by the newly appointed Director-General of the I.M.S., George Bomford. 'Captain Liston has views about the causation of plague which he has never had an opportunity of working out thoroughly', wrote Bomford. 'The flea theory seems to me to be very promising. I would therefore agree to the deputation of Captain Liston.'[110]

Liston was thus able over the next few years to develop the work which he had begun under the jealous eye of Haffkine. In particular, he was able to continue investigation into the peculiar method by which the rat-flea preserved plague bacilli, over some days, in its gizzard, and allowed them to multiply, only to inject them into those from whom it drew blood. Liston's work on the mechanism of plague transmission was completed, in England, by Martin and Arthur Bacot. But it was Liston who had undoubtedly pointed the way.[111] By 1910 he was in charge of continuing investigation in India, on behalf of the Plague Advisory Committee, into many aspects of the disease.[112] By 1910, too, the results of the well-funded studies by Liston and his co-workers were being published in special 'Plague Supplements' of the *Journal of Hygiene*, lavishly produced by the Cambridge University Press.[113] These studies are still frequently quoted in the scientific literature. Certainly so far as plague was concerned medical research in India had begun by 1910 to take on a distinctly twentieth-century appearance – so very different from the floundering, and indeed, the muddle, of less than fifteen years before.[114] By 1910, too, the rat-flea theory of plague causation was largely accepted in the circles of the Indian Medical Service. For that matter, it was by this time also largely accepted by the Indian Civil Service. At first sight it would seem as though, at last, the 'scientific' and the 'medical' had triumphed over the 'political', the 'imperial'. But was this altogether the case?

We cannot entirely neglect the role of that great imperialist viceroy Lord Curzon in the minor scientific take-off that appears to have occurred in India in the early years of this century. Longer-term civil servant initiative in India, it is true, seems to have been even more important,[115] although Curzon was probably to some extent responsible for a change in the processes of selection that made it possible for George Bomford, who was certainly not the most senior person available, to come to the headship of the I.M.S. in 1905.[116] In any case, whether such initiatives were primarily viceregal or primarily bureaucratic they were still basically 'political'.

But it is now becoming clear that much of the initiative for an increase in the amount of scientific work in India was not coming from within that country. It was not coming from the I.M.S., nor even from the I.C.S. It had its origin, rather, in the centre of empire, London. 'Advisory committees' of the Royal Society played their part, as Professor Roy MacLeod has shown.[117] The India Office made a contribution, too – certainly in the case of plague research. But one is forced to conclude that the major initiative in the creation of an ethos in the metropolitan centre which was favourable to research in tropical medicine came not from the India Office but from the Colonial Office.

Joseph Chamberlain is popularly given the credit for the growth of Colonial Office interest in tropical medicine, although, as in the case of Curzon in India, the role of the civil servant seems in fact to have been greater than that of the man at the top.[118] In any case it is quite apparent that by 1904 there was frequent contact in London between representatives of the Royal Society, the Lister Institute, the India Office and the Colonial Office – with the Colonial Office generally taking the lead. It was from such contacts – particularly, one suspects, in connection with the Tropical Diseases Research Fund[119] – that the Plague Advisory Committee appears to have arisen. These Colonial Office initiatives doubtless permitted members of the Colonial Medical Service – the service to which the somewhat hapless Dr Lowson from Hong Kong had belonged – to hold their heads a good deal higher in the presence of the Indian Medical Service. Such were the ironies of imperialism.

Of course, the India Office and the Colonial Office did not interest themselves in tropical medicine primarily for altruistic reasons, although such motives were not entirely absent. The British government contributions to the financing of the newly founded London and Liverpool Schools of Tropical Medicine, especially through the Tropical Diseases Research Fund, were largely an expression of a desire to make the tropics safe for Europeans. 'Permanence' was to be made possible. The 'tools of empire' were being tempered, refashioned, largely – certainly so far as the Colonial Office was concerned – for the benefit of the imperial power.

One final point needs to be added. It is by no means clear that the considerable development of research on plague in India in the first and second decades of this century was to any great extent responsible for the alleviation of the lot of ordinary Indians – plague victims and their relatives. Knowledge of the causes of plague did not, in spite of the Lister Institute's high hopes in 1904, lead to a rapid reduction in the extent of plague in India. Plague began to diminish in India in the 1920s and 1930s, in part, perhaps, because of an increased knowledge of the ways in which plague could travel in merchandise[120] (a knowledge which, incidentally, had it been available in 1897, could have made a good deal of difference to the deliberations of the Venice Sanitary Conference). But it seems likely that plague in India began to diminish primarily because rats and other similar creatures were beginning to breed immune. Possibly, too, there were changes in the 'virulence', the pathogenicity, of the plague bacillus itself.[121] DDT for the rats and their fleas, and streptomycin and the like for the human victims, eventually did make a difference. But that was not until the 1940s and 1950s. By that time plague had already gone into a fairly steep decline in India. Prior to the 1940s, so far as plague was concerned, India remained basically at the mercy of the vast impersonal demographic forces that the *Annalistes* are perpetually emphasising,[122] and in fact there was very little that either the practitioners of western medicine, or the officials, could do about it. Until the 1940s, it could be argued, plague in India might well have been better left to the *hakims* and the *vaids*.

Notes

Abbreviations used:

BG	*Bombay Gazette*
D/O	Demi-official
encl.	enclosed
GOI	Government of India
IOL	India Office Library, London
IOR	India Office Records, London
KW	Keep-with
NAI	National Archives of India, New Delhi
PP	Parliamentary Papers, Great Britain
PRO	Public Record Office, London
Progs	Proceedings
TI	*Times of India Overland Weekly/Weekly Mail Edition*
UPSA	Uttar Pradesh State Archives, Lucknow
WBSA	West Bengal State Archives, Calcutta

1 See *BG*, late-September–mid-October 1896; Telegram, Viceroy to Secretary of State for India, 30 September 1896, *Papers relating to Bubonic Plague in India . . . up to March 1897*, p. 3, PP 1897 (C.8386), lxiii.
2 Letter, 'Another I.M.S. Officer', *TI*, 2 September 1899.
3 *BG*, 5 October 1896; Lord Sandhurst, Governor, Bombay, to Lord Elgin, Viceroy, 2 October 1897, Elgin Papers, MSS. Eur. F84/71, IOL.
4 *BG*, 1 October 1896.
5 *Ibid.*
6 *Ibid.*, 12 October 1896.
7 *The Bombay Plague, being a History of the Progress of Plague in the Bombay Presidency from September 1896 to June 1899.* Compiled by Captain J. K. Condon, Government of Bombay, 1900, p. 125.
8 *TI*, 12 February 1898.
9 F. G. Hutchins, *The Illusion of Permanence: British Imperialism in India*, Princeton, N.J., 1967.
10 D. R. Headrick, *The Tools of Empire: Technology and European Imperialism in the Nineteenth Century*, New York, 1981.
11 See, e.g., I. J. Catanach, 'Plague and the Indian village', in P. Robb (ed.), *Rural India: Land, Power and Society under British Rule*, London, 1983, esp. p. 216; D. Arnold, 'Touching the body: perspectives on the Indian plague, 1896–1900', in R. Guha (ed.), *Subaltern Studies*, V, Delhi, 1987, pp. 55-90.
12 Cf., e.g., L. Chevalier (ed.), *Le Choléra: La Première Épidémie du Xix[e] Siècle*, La

Roche-sur-Yon, 1958; A. Briggs, 'Cholera and society in the nineteenth century', *Past and Present*, 19, 1961, pp. 76-96. See also I. J. Catanach, 'Rats, lice and Indian history', in J. McGuire et al (eds.), *Problems and Methods of Enquiry in South Asian History*, Centre for South and Southeast Asian Studies, University of Western Australia, 1984, pp. 55-70.

13 *BG*, 13 January 1897; see also *TI*, 26 February 1898.

14 L. Rogers, 'The incidence and spread of cholera in India: forecasting and control of epidemics', *Indian Medical Research Memoirs*, IX, 1928, p. 4.

15 *Minutes of Evidence taken by the Indian Plague Commission with Appendices*, III, pp. 361-7, esp. Q.26722, PP 1900 (Cd.141), xxxii.

16 D. G. Crawford, *A History of the Indian Medical Service, 1600–1913*, 2 vols., London and Calcutta, 1914; R. Jeffery, 'Allopathic medicine: a case of deprofessionalization', *Economic and Political Weekly*, Bombay, XIII, 21 January 1978, pp. 101-13; T. J. Johnson and M. Caygill, 'The British Medical Association and its overseas branches: a short history', *Journal of Imperial and Commonwealth History*, I, 1973, pp. 303-29.

17 J. C. Hume Jr., 'Medicine in the Punjab 1848–1911; ethnicity and professionalization in the control of an occupation', unpublished Ph.D. diss., Duke University, 1977.

18 *Ibid.*, chapter III.

19 *Ibid.*, p. 93.

20 *Plague Commission, Mins of Ev.*, I, Q. 7773, PP 1900 (Cd.139), xxx.

21 Secretary of State to Governor, Bombay, 18 January 1897, *Papers relating to Bubonic Plague*, p. 5.

22 Sir E. Monson to Marquess of Salisbury, Paris, 7 February 1897, PRO M.H. 19/239.

23 Jean-Noël Biraben, 'Certain demographic characteristics of the plague epidemic in France, 1720–22', *Daedalus*, XLVII, 1968, pp. 536-45.

24 L. F. Hirst, *The Conquest of Plague. A Study of the Evolution of Epidemiology*, Oxford, 1953, pp. 105-6.

25 N. Howard-Jones, *The Scientific Background of the International Sanitary Conferences 1851–1938*, Geneva, 1975.

26 Arthur Godley (Permanent Under-Secretary, India Office) to Cleghorn, 9 February 1897, encl. Godley to Foreign Office, 12 February 1897, PRO M.H. 19/239. Many of the most important papers on the Venice Conference are in this collection; see also PRO F.O. 83/1573 and 1574, IOR L/E/7/391.

27 Memo by 'H.F.', Foreign Office, 5 December 1897, encl. Secretary of State to Viceroy, Revenue Despatch 22 of 10 February 1898, Enclosure 2. Bengal Municipal (Medical) Progs, May 1898, 96, IOR.

28 The most lavish of these reports (4 vols. bound in red and gold, found today in many libraries around the world) is *The Plague in India, 1896, 1897*, compiled by R. Nathan, GOI, Simla, 1898.

29 D. Arnold, 'Cholera and colonialism in British India', *Past and Present*, 113, 1986, esp. p. 29; Arnold, 'Smallpox and colonial medicine in nineteenth-century India' (in this volume).

30 Anil Seal, 'Imperialism and nationalism in India', in J. Gallagher, G. Johnson and A. Seal (eds.), *Locality, Province and Nation: Essays on Indian Politics 1870–1940*, Cambridge, 1973, p. 9.

31 Harcourt Butler to his sister Margaret, 27 April 1897, Butler Papers, MSS. Eur. F116/5, IOL.

32 *Plague Commission, Mins. of Ev.*, III, Q.17194.

33 *Correspondence Relative to the Outbreak of Plague at Hong Kong*, PP 1894 (C.7461), lvii; *Further Correspondence Relative to the Outbreak of Bubonic Plague at Hong Kong*, PP 1894 (C.7545), lvii.

34 James A. Lowson, *Report on the Epidemic of Plague from 22nd February to 16th July 1897*, [London], 1897, p. 45.

35 Elgin to Lord George Hamilton, 25 May 1897, Hamilton Papers, MSS. Eur. D509/5, IOL.

36 See W. W. Beveridge, 'Medical report on the plague in Poona', in M. E. Couchman (ed.), *Supplement to the Account of Plague Administration in the Bombay Presi-*

dency from September 1896 to May 1897, Government of Bombay, 1897.

37 *BG*, 29 March 1897.

38 On this episode see I. J. Catanach, 'Poona politicians and the plague', *South Asia*, N.S., VII, 1984, pp. 1-18; and Arnold, 'Touching the body'.

39 See the *Englishman* (Calcutta), January–July 1897; also J & P 1896A in L/PJ/6/456, IOR, especially Elgin to Sir Antony MacDonnell, 6 July 1897 and MacDonnell to Elgin, D/O of 16 July 1897.

40 Cf. T. R. Metcalf, 'The British and the moneylender in nineteenth-century India', *Journal of Modern History*, XXXIV, 1962, pp. 394 and 397; also Metcalf, *The Aftermath of Revolt: India 1857–1870*, Princeton, N.J., 1964, esp. p. 323.

41 Letters from R. A. Lamb (Collector, Poona) and 'Justitia', *TI*, 3 September 1897; also *TI*, 6 August 1897 (editorial), and 27 August 1897 ('Notes of the Week').

42 *TI*, 12 August 1899, ('Notes of the Week').

43 Reade to Godley, 3 March 1898, Kilbracken Papers, MSS. Eur. F102/6, IOL.

44 Mrs Edythe Lutzker of New York assisted me in my work on Haffkine, as she has assisted others. See her entry on Haffkine, *Dictionary of Scientific Biography*, VI New York, 1972. See also Mark Popovsky, *The Story of Dr Haffkine*, trans. V. Vezey, Moscow [1964]; Selman A. Waksman, *The Brilliant and Tragic Life of W. M. W. Haffkine*, New Brunswick, N.J., 1964.

45 The question as to whether Haffkine was the first to discover this technique is discussed in G. H. Bornside, 'Waldemar Haffkine's cholera vaccines and the Ferran–Haffkine priority dispute', *Journal of the History of Medicine*, XXXVII, 1982, pp. 399-422; and, earlier, in W. Bullock's somewhat unfavourable obituary of Haffkine, *Journal of Pathology and Bacteriology*, XXXIV, 1931, pp. 125-9.

46 Bullock, obituary of Haffkine, p. 128; Popovsky, *Haffkine*, pp. 71-2; Waksman, *Haffkine*, p. 21. See also *TI* (quoting the *Pioneer*), 4 June 1898.

47 Reginald Gilbert, letter to editor, *Englishman*, 11 May 1898; *TI*, 10 September 1898 (editorial); J. Pollen (I.C.S. retired), letter to editor, *TI*, 20 April 1907; Popovsky, *Haffkine*, pp. 102-3.

48 Bainbridge to Private Secretary, Governor, Bombay, D/O 'Strictly Confidential' of 19 January 1898; Elgin to Sandhurst, Confidential, 7 February 1898 (from which it emerges that the GOI was 'on the point of' commending inoculation when the Bombay controversy blew up). MSS. Eur. F84/125K, IOL.

49 Elgin to Sandhurst, 19 March 1898.

50 Popovsky, *Haffkine*, pp. 64, 74.

51 Obituary of Simpson, *Nature*, 24 October 1931, pp. 695-6.

52 For Simpson's activities as Health Officer, Calcutta, see C. Furedy, 'Whose responsibility? Dilemmas of Calcutta's bustee policy in the nineteenth century', *South Asia*, N.S., V, 1982, pp. 38-9.

53 *History and Proceedings of the Bengal Plague Commission 1896 to 1898*, Government of Bengal, 1899, pp. 2-8; on disapproval in the Viceroy's circle of the activities of the Board see Sir John Woodburn (Home Member) to Elgin, D/O of 20 February 1897, MSS. Eur. F84/70, IOL.

54 On the close relationships at this time between export-orientated European business in Calcutta and the Government of Bengal (though not the Government of India) see R. Ray, *Urban Roots of Indian Nationalism: Pressure Groups and Conflict of Interests in Calcutta City Politics, 1875–1939*, New Delhi, 1979. D. F. Mackenzie, a partner in the firm of Burn & Co. and representative of the Bengal Chamber of Commerce in the Bengal Legislative Council, was a brother of the Lieutenant-Governor, Sir Alexander Mackenzie (*ibid.*, p. 56). On the Calcutta Municipal Act see C. Furedy, 'Lord Curzon and the reform of the Calcutta Corporation: a case-study in imperial decision-making', *South Asia*, N.S., I, 1978, pp. 75-87.

55 Risley to Secretary, Home Department, GOI, 1014 Medical, of 24 February 1897, Bengal Municipal (Medical) Progs, March 1897, 34, File 2-P/6 196, WBSA.

56 *TI*, 26 April 1898, quoted Revenue Sanitary Letter from India 11 of 12 May 1898, enclosure 67, IOR.

57 See MacDonnell's letters to Elgin, January–June 1897, especially 16 February and 9

May, MSS. Eur. F84/70, IOL; also G.A.D., File 449C/1900 (Box 12), UPSA.

58 *Civil and Military Gazette,* 10 April 1898.

59 R. H. [Harvey], 'Note on Plague Administration', 18 April 1898, in R & S 2186/1898, L/E/7/408, IOR. See also GOI Home Sanitary A Progs, August 1898, 777-813, and KWs, NAI.

60 F. N. White, 'Twenty years of plague in India with special reference to the outbreak of 1917–18', *Indian Journal of Medical Research,* VI, 1918–19, p. 191; see also Catanach, 'Rats, lice and Indian history', pp. 62-4.

61 Memorandum embodying the Conclusions of the Conference at Simla in June 1898, and other papers in IOR L/E/7/408.

62 G.A.D., File 486C of 1900, UPSA; GOI Home Public A Progs, June 1900, 291-302, B Progs, August 1900, 133, NAI; MacDonnell to Curzon, 24 April 1900, Curzon Papers, MSS. F111/201, pt. i, IOL.

63 GOI Revenue Sanitary Letter 12 of 28 August 1902, IOR.

64 Memorandum embodying the Conclusions. . . (see note 61 above).

65 Hewett, Note, 28 July 1898, E. [Elgin], Notes, 6 and 17 August 1898, GOI Home Sanitary A Progs, August 1898, KW1, NAI. Elgin was wary of criticism of plague administration developing along lines similar to the criticism of famine administration in Bombay which had come from a recent official inquiry.

66 Lister to Godley, 24 September 1905, R & S 2186/1898, IOR L/E/7/408.

67 Godley to Lister, 28 September 1898, MSS. Eur. F102/1, IOL.

68 *TI,* 12 November 1898, 'Notes of the Week'.

69 Professor T. R. Fraser; born Calcutta 1841 but displayed considerable ignorance of the Indian situation, and to the end maintained that the basic problem was one of sanitation.

70 Dr Armand Ruffer. On the Egyptian administration's hostility to plague inoculation see *TI,* 30 July 1897 (editorial), 5 November 1898 and 9 September 1899.

71 L. Colebrook, 'Almroth Edward Wright', *Obituary Notices of Fellows of the Royal Society,* VI, November 1948, pp. 297-309.

72 *Report of the Indian Plague Commission with Appendices and Summary,* chapter IV, PP 1902 (Cd.810), lxxii.

73 *Plague Commission Report,* pp. 278 *et seq.* However the Commission did hold (p. 370) that serum therapy as applied to plague was 'nonetheless the only method which holds forth a prospect of ultimate success.'

74 *Annales de l'Institut Pasteur,* October 1898.

75 *Plague Commission Report,* pp. 75-7.

76 Waksman, *Haffkine,* pp. 39-41; P. A. Dalal, 'The last epidemic of plague in Bombay. (A forgotten chapter in the history of the city)', *Indian Practitioner,* October 1959, p. 932.

77 T. S. Kuhn, *The Structure of Scientific Revolutions,* Chicago, 1964. Cf. David Arnold on 'medical mind-sets', in his review of Donald R. Hopkins, *Princes and Peasants: Smallpox in History,* in *Peasant Studies,* XIII, 1986, p. 130.

78 R. Harvey, 'Note on Plague Commission's Report as to "Plague Measures"', 21 June 1900, GOI Home Sanitary (Plague) A Progs, July 1900, 244-52, NAI.

79 W. M. Haffkine, 'Concerning inoculation against plague and pneumonia and the experimental study of curative methods', *Journal of Hygiene,* XV, 1915–17, p. 65 and n. 1; *Dictionary of Scientific Biography,* XV, New York, 1976.

80 Haffkine, 'Concerning inoculation', p. 76; on Wright and the 'flea' theory see below p. 163 and note 107.

81 *Plague Commission Report,* p. 409.

82 'A', letter to editor, *Pioneer,* 15 March 1902. Cf. *TI,* 13 October 1906, on 'The Poona Season': 'Familiarity breeds contempt, and although plague is increasing in the Cantonment and environs, but little heed is taken of it now, whereas a few years ago it would have caused a panic.'

83 The Punjab government claimed that plague inoculation had proved itself in the success of an inoculation programme in the Punjab in the period since the Plague Commission report had been written. See *The History of Plague in the Punjab, with* a Memo. of the Measures adopted for dealing with it and Instructions regarding the Measures to be adopted in 1902–3 [Punjab Plague Manual, 1902], chapter III. For Rivaz's concern, on another occasion, for quick results that would enhance his reputation, see N. G. Barrier, 'The Punjab disturbances of 1907: the response of the British government in India to agrarian unrest', *Modern Asian Studies*, I, 1967, p. 366.

84 E. Wilkinson, *Report on Plague and Inoculation in the Punjab from October 1st 1902 to September 30th 1903. . .*, Government of Punjab, 1904, p. 48.

85 W. S. Marris, Note, 9 August 1903, on GOI Home Sanitary (Plague) Deposit Progs, October 1903, 2-4, NAI.

86 Wilkinson, *Punjab Plague Report 1902–3*, pp. 46-8.

87 See letter from Ronald Ross and others, *The Times*, 29 July 1907.

88 Wilkinson, *Punjab Plague Report 1902–3*, Punjab Government Review of Report, p. 11.

89 (Dr) E. Taylor to (Surgeon-Major) W. B. Bannerman, D/O of 15 November 1902, encl. Haffkine to Risley, Officiating Secretary, Home Department, GOI, D/O 310 of 10 February 1903 (Enclosure 51 with GOI Finance and Commerce Letter 144 of 12 May 1904, R & S 1703/1903, IOR L/E/7/486).

90 Haffkine, evidence, Jenkins Commission Minutes of Evidence, p. 21. GOI Home Sanitary (Plague) A Progs, April 1903, 1-62, NAI.

91 Risley, Note, 13 December 1902, Progs cited, 34.

92 Progs cited, note 90 above.

93 At least according to Sir Arthur Hirtzel, as interpreted by Dietmar Rothermund, 'Emancipation or re-integration. The politics of Gopal Krishna Gokhale and Herbert Hope Risley', in D. A. Low (ed.), *Soundings in Modern South Asian History*, London, 1968, p. 143.

94 Risley, Note, 9 March 1903 on Progs cited, note 90 above.

95 Lord Lamington, Governor, Bombay, to Secretary of State for India, 21 June 1906, Lamington Letter Books, Duke University Library (Micro 675, IOL).

96 Risley, Note, 9 March 1903 (see note 94 above). The first report of the Jenkins Commission is in the NAI collection cited note 90; the second is in GOI Home Sanitary (Plague) A Progs, November 1903, 11-25, NAI.

97 *The Times*, 29 July 1907; see also Ronald Ross's letter, *The Times*, 15 March 1907, and Dalal, 'The last epidemic of plague', p. 951.

98 Butler, 'Note to His Honour', 25 April 1904, on P. Gray, Commissioner, Lucknow Division, to Inspector-General of Civil Hospitals, U.P., 1115/XXVII – 173 of 1 March 1904, U.P. Sanitary File 775B of 1903, UPSA.

99 J. Chaytor-White, Chief Plague Officer, on Mirzapur District, Plague Administration in the United Provinces for the Year 1903, File cited, UPSA.

100 J.R.D.S. [Dunlop Smith], Note on Plague, 24 June 1907, Morley Papers, MSS. Eur. D 573/12, IOL.

101 Cf. Catanach, '"Fatalism"?'. See also D. Arnold, 'Gramsci and peasant subalternity in India', *Journal of Peasant Studies*, XI 1984, esp. p. 169; for some very interesting hints about Indian concepts of 'crisis' see P. Greenough, 'The death of an uncrowned king – C. R. Das and political crisis in twentieth-century Bengal', *Comparative Studies in Society and History*, XXVIII, 1986, esp. pp. 414-20.

102 J. Ashburton Thompson, *Report of the Board of Health on a Second Outbreak of Plague at Sydney, 1902*, Sydney, Government Printer, New South Wales, 1902, pp. 2, 70; and (for reports by Tidswell) pp. 67-8, 71-4. Here I should like to thank Dr Peter Paisley, of Sydney, for a copy of his unpublished paper, 'Sydney and the Plague'. On Elkington see *Australian Dictionary of Biography*, VIII, Melbourne, 1981.

103 See M. Roe, 'The establishment of the Australian Department of Health: its background and significance', *Historical Studies*, XVII, 1976, esp. p. 189.

104 W. M. Haffkine, *Summarised Report on the Bombay Plague Research Laboratory, for 1896–1902*, Government of Bombay, 1903, p. 34.

105 J. S. C. Elkington, 'Fleas and plague convection', *Australasian Medical Gazette*, 20 August 1903, p. 352.

106 W. Glen Liston, 'Plague, rats and fleas. (Read before the Bombay Natural History Society, on 24th November 1904)', *Indian Medical Gazette*, XLI, February 1905, pp. 43-9. Liston there claims to have published an earlier paper on the subject in the (revived?) *Transactions of the Bombay Medical and Physical Society* in February 1903, but I have been unable to find this. See also Liston, 'The Milroy Lectures on Plague', *British Medical Journal*, 1924, pp. 900-3, 950-4, 997-1001; Dalal, 'The last epidemic of plague', p. 934; obituary of Liston, *Lancet*, 25 November 1950, p. 657.

107 The whole sad story of Liston's relations with Haffkine is documented in GOI Home Sanitary (Plague) Letter 18 of 12 November 1903 and enclosures, IOR; see also R & S 3073/1903, IOR L/E/7/486. On Wright's encouragement of Liston see obituary of Liston noted note 106 above and Dalal, 'The last epidemic of plague', p. 934.

108 On Martin see H. Chick, 'Charles James Martin', *Biographical Memoirs of Fellows of the Royal Society*, II, 1956, pp. 173-208, esp. p. 175 on the way the 'Martin spirit' lived on in Australian medicine.

109 H. Chick, M. Hume and M. Macfarlane, *War on Disease: A History of the Lister Institute*, London, 1971, pp. 95-7.

110 Bomford, Note, 4 February 1905, on GOI Home Sanitary (Plague) A Progs, August 1905, 12, NAI.

111 Chick et al, *War on Disease*, pp. 100-2; Liston, *British Medical Journal*, 31 May 1924, p. 954; C.J.M. [Martin], obituary of Bacot, *Nature*, 13 May 1922, pp. 618-20.

112 See, e.g., Liston to Hewett, Lieutenant-Governor, United Provinces, 27 May 1910; Liston to Hewett, 5 September 1910; UP Sanitary File 115/10 of 1911, UPSA.

113 The Plague Supplements published by the *Journal of Hygiene* between 1906 and 1914 were republished as *Reports on Plague Investigations in India. Issued by the Advisory Committee appointed by the Secretary of State for India, the Royal Society and the Lister Institute of Preventive Medicine*, [I], Cambridge, 1912, and II, pt. i, Cambridge, 1914.

114 See, e.g., 'Sir Leonard Rogers', *Dictionary of National Biography, 1961-1970*, Oxford, 1981; Sir John Boyd, 'Leonard Rogers', *Biographical Memoirs of Fellows of the Royal Society*, IX, 1963, esp. p. 265.

115 Cf. I. J. Catanach, *Rural Credit in Western India: Rural Credit and the Co-operative Movement in the Bombay Presidency, 1875-1930*, Berkeley, 1970, pp. 36-8 and note 100; E. R. Bonner, 'The economic policy of the Government of India, 1898–1905', unpublished M.A. thesis, University of London, 1955, remains of use in this matter.

116 'Government acted on the principle of promotion by selection to a greater extent than had ever been done before' in 'promoting *a* Lieut.-Colonel S. G. Bomford'. Crawford, *Indian Medical Service*, II, p. 41. (My italics.)

117 R. M. MacLeod, 'Scientific advice for British India', *Modern Asian Studies*, IX, 1975, pp. 343-84.

118 R. V. Kubicek, *The Administration of Imperialism: Joseph Chamberlain at the Colonial Office*, Durham, N.C., 1969, pp. 14, 20, 178 and (especially) chapter VII.

119 See *Report of the Advisory Committee for the Tropical Diseases Research Fund of the Year 1906*, PP 1907 (Cd.3306), lxviii, 639.

120 See F. N. White, Report on Plague in Rawalpindi City, 9 August 1917, pp. 8-9, GOI Education (Sanitary) B Progs, August 1917, 23, NAI; White, 'Twenty years of plague', pp. 209-10, 216.

121 White, Sanitary Commissioner with the Government of India in 1919, noted ('Twenty years of plague', p. 215) the decreasing virulence of plague but admitted that this could 'in no wise be attributed to the increasing efficiency of our plague measures'. He put forward the possibility of rats breeding immune. See also Catanach, 'Rats, lice and Indian history', p. 62-4.

122 See, e.g., E. Le Roy Ladurie, 'Motionless history', *Social Science History*, I, 1977, p. 133.

CHAPTER EIGHT

The influenza pandemic in Southern Rhodesia: a crisis of comprehension

Terence Ranger

The influenza pandemic of 1918 is no subject for a triumphalist medical history. No effective treatment was available at the time, and the influenza viruses still defy medical science.[1] Hence those historians of empire who have published work on the pandemic have not discussed diagnosis or cure but focused rather on its demographic consequences,[2] or its disruption of colonial labour management,[3] or its stimulus to programmes of public health.[4] These are all important questions, but it is the aim of this chapter to address another about which little has yet been published – the influenza pandemic as a conceptual crisis, as a challenge to existing explanations of affliction. This is a question to which researchers are increasingly paying attention.

Howard Phillips' doctoral thesis for the University of Cape Town contains a fascinating chapter on 'popular and religious explanations' of the pandemic, which draws on much material from white and some from black sources. Luke Williams of La Trobe University is embarking on similar research on the impact of the pandemic in Nigeria.[5] But it seems likely that this chapter will be the first published discussion of the topic. Focusing exclusively on black intellectual history, it argues that in Southern Rhodesia all the available resources of western and indigenous medicine and ideology were drawn upon in an attempt to explain and contain the pandemic. None of them succeeded in containing it. Despite this, adherents of both western and indigenous medicine and religion were able to persuade themselves that their chosen system of ideas had succeeded in explaining it. Nevertheless, for many other Africans the failures of 1918 called for new types of explanation and practice. When these new types emerged, breaking with both indigenous and colonial ideologies, they legitimated themselves by reference back to the pandemic of 1918.

Respectable scholarship has played down the melodrama of the 1918 pandemic. For my purpose I need to play it up. Unless we can grasp the influenza epidemic as crisis we cannot understand its impact on ideas. So in the first part of this chapter I briefly trace how influenza spread in Southern Rhodesia in 1918; where its impact was most dramatically felt; and how that drama was recounted and remembered. In the second part of the chapter I describe the range of responses to the pandemic by the Native Department, by government doctors, by employers and by missionaries. I shall then go on in a third section to show that most Africans regarded these European responses as at worst murderous and at best irrelevant. Even those Africans most attracted to European medicine could place little confidence in it in October and November 1918. Africans meanwhile drew on a whole range of indigenous techniques and explanations in an attempt to deal with the influenza themselves. Some had recourse to herbal remedies. Others turned to diviners in order to detect the witches who had brought the disease; or to emissaries from the cave-cult of the High God; or to prophets of new spirits which had announced their arrival by means of the pandemic. Despite the universality and scale of the pandemic, these particular indigenous explanations were evidently convincing to many. But some Africans came to feel that none of them, nor western medicine, had been adequate to deal with influenza. In a fourth and final section of the chapter I argue that the influenza crisis partly gave rise to, and more largely legitimated, new movements of explanation, which prohibited the use of both western and traditional medicines.

The spread and impact of the influenza pandemic

The influenza epidemic broke out among Southern Rhodesian Africans wherever they were clustered together and at the same time in contact with travellers. In the two large towns – Salisbury and Bulawayo – a major mechanism in spreading the disease was the symbolically appropriate Pass Office, to which all black applicants for employment had to report. Outside the towns, influenza raged most spectacularly in the mining compounds, where hundreds of African miners were gathered together, in ramshackle housing, fed on very poor rations, and the objects of authoritarian medical treatment. In districts where there were no towns or mines, influenza first became apparent in mission boarding schools, and in districts where there were no schools it first became apparent at the Native Commissioner's headquarters. This pattern of incidence meant that Africans naturally connected the disease with the operation of the colonial economy. When in November 1918 some mining companies planned to send out patrols to round up African workers who had fled from the diseased compounds so that production could again commence, Chief Native Commissioner Taylor warned that 'the natives have an idea that the Europeans are responsible for the introduction of the disease and any reference to labour matters at the present time might have the effect of defeating our present object which is to calm the natives'.[6] Eventually the disease was carried almost everywhere as men ran away from the towns and compounds.

The death rate was highest and the impact most dramatic in the mining compounds. The Chilimanzi district report for October 1918 recorded 300 deaths at Falcon Mine alone. 'About 100 natives were picked up in the Township by cart from a house to house collection and in the streets and were buried in the same trenches . . . Several hundreds deserted from the mine.' The deserters left a trail of dead and dying men. 'Dead natives are lying on the road . . . Many dead bodies are reported lying on the Central Estates and also the Rhodesdale Estate.'[7] These bare official details were later fleshed out in all their horror by the radical missionary Arthur Shearly Cripps who had collected oral testimonies immediately after the pandemic. These testimonies spoke of 'the sickness that was newly come upon the mine boys, as if the spirits of the dead – every spirit that had not found its rest – had come to one place, and would never cease from anger'. They remembered with horror the death carts and the mass burials:

> It was dreadful. They brought them in a cart, the dead with their stiff feet pushed forth from their blankets . . . They cast them out into a great pit. Some had blankets and some wore loincloths. But there was one little boy . . . as naked as he was born . . . In the evening we ran away, after they had taken our sick brother to the Hospital. We said, 'He will die tonight. Motsobo will die. Then they will put him under the iron roof in the house of the dead near the Hospital gate. And tomorrow when another pit has been dug, the cart will come, and they will take him away to sleep in that pit, where none has his own bed, but all lie together and trouble one another and not one of them has rest.' . . . We were so frightened that before the sun set we had run away . . . We followed the iron way that the steamer trains followed until we came to an old train carriage which had been left by the road. . . When we climbed in we saw a dead man's stiff feet stretched forth in the doorway, and we screamed and threw ourselves down.[8]

It was generally agreed that the incidence of the disease and the death rate were lower in the rural areas, where women and young children were the main victims. Nevertheless, reports by missionaries who worked in the rural areas were alarming enough. The Anglican R. H. Baker, of Penhalonga mission in eastern Manicaland, described an expedition into the neighbouring Reserves. Some homesteads had no cases of flu; others quite nearby were universally afflicted. In one 'nearly everyone was sick . . . twelve people were there and one was lying dead. The father of the family, who was alright, had gone to dig a grave, taking with him a boy who was just ailing. All the rest were sick.' Baker came across fugitives from the mines, lying either in shelters built for them away from the homesteads or dead 'by the wayside'. He illustrated the way in which the disease could strike with terrible suddenness by a 'most pathetic' story of a mother who had gone to collect her sick children from school and who on the way home 'as they were going through a pass between two mountains, . . . fell down and died by the wayside'.[9]

The sudden onset of the disease, the bodies left lying unburied, the fate of whole homesteads – all left their mark on the rural imagination. I discovered in 1981 when I was carrying out fieldwork in Makoni district, which lies some two-thirds of the way between Harare and Mutare, that the Bvekerwa clan, who claim descent from Ndafunya, Chief Makoni at the time of the pandemic, still call their place of residence Nyahonye, 'the place of worms', because so many had died there of influenza in 1918. The Native Commissioner, Makoni, calculated that 3 per cent of the African population of his district had died of flu in 1918. Anglican missionaries in Makoni thought it was 10 per cent. In Matabeleland death rates in the mines, as given in district reports, varied between 15 per cent and 6 per cent; for the rural areas they varied from 1 per cent to 3.6 per cent. These rural estimates were almost certainly too low, since very many child deaths went unreported and unremarked. Children born during the epidemic who did survive could carry the given name 'Influenza' through the rest of their lives. In October 1918 itself a whole series of local names for the disease sprang up, each seeking to encapsulate its dire identity. In central Matabeleland, 'with their usual aptness in nomenclature they named the disease "malibuzwe" (Let enquiries be made concerning it), ironically suggesting that, all being prostrated alike, no mutual, neighbourly inquiries as to health could be made'.[10]

European responses to the pandemic

European reactions to the outbreak of flu among Africans were varied. In the towns the chief response was fear of contagion. Stephen Thornton, the foremost social historian of Bulawayo, writes that 'the 'flu epidemic in 1918 brought as much terror to the European population as the outbreak of the Revolt twenty years previously'. In the long term this terror led to public health recommendations from an Influenza Committee. In the short term it led to an attempt strictly to isolate sick Africans in the Bulawayo lazaretto. Africans dreaded this confinement. The lazaretto had been condemned in 1914 as merely 'a shed, entirely unsuited for the treatment of disease'. Sick Africans did everything they could to avoid being sent there. Gibson Tawako of the Northern Rhodesian Bantu Association wrote complaining to the Bulawayo Town Clerk in October 1918 that Africans were offered no help except this odious isolation: 'We feel that more help should be done. We saw boys sitting down by the Presbyterian Church; we asked them why they were sitting down there; the reply was, we are sick and afraid of staying in the location unless we be sent to the Lazaretto.'[11] Nevertheless, some 800 sufferers were 'removed to the lazaretto for treatment' by the Medical Officer of Health, who just had time to note that Africans had 'an instinctive dislike' of the institution before he fell sick himself, along with most of the African municipal employees who were supposed to guard the place. Seizing their opportunity the sick and dying broke out of confinement – 'a large number of native sufferers fled from the lazaretto and spread the disease far and wide'. As they fled they took the ill repute of the Bulawayo lazaretto with them, so that administrative officers and doctors visiting homesteads in rural Matabeleland had to assuage fears of 'being taken to Bulawayo for hospital treatment' before people would admit to the disease.[12] The same pattern was repeated in Mashonaland and Manicaland, where sick Africans fled from the Salisbury and Umtali lazarettos. In Makoni district, between Salisbury and Umtali, the first cases of rural influenza were 'kept so secret by the natives at first that it was impossible to locate. This secrecy appeared due to their fear of being brought into lazarettes about which the most gruesome stories were current.'[13]

Africans had no more confidence in the 'hospitals' at mining compounds and hardly any attempts to isolate sufferers succeeded. The only success, at German Mine in Belingwe, was itself a classic example of authoritarianism. There the whole African population of 200 – workers, servants, women, children – were totally quarantined in the compound before the disease had reached them. The Native Commissioner instructed the police 'boys' and boss 'boys' of the mine to prevent any movement in or out. 'They asked me what power they had to enforce the order and I suggested they should use their sjamboks in moderation.'[14]

In the rural areas Europeans were less concerned with contagion or with coercion. The Native Department at first feared widespread unrest and then feared a collapse of agricultural activity. Gradually, however, especially as mission stations and schools recovered from their early dose of the 'flu and began to send out parties of 'salted' converts to help sufferers in the Reserves, a humanitarian note was sounded. Some optimistic missionaries believed that the pandemic was a God-given opportunity to win Africans over by effective loving-kindness and to compensate in the countryside for the scarring experience of the towns. It might even have been so had the whites possessed an effective remedy. But it is clear that the medicines with which administrators, employers and missionaries began to dose Africans were idiosyncratic to a degree. In Inyanga the Native Commissioner found 'quinine and epsom salts very effective'; in Melsetter a mass inoculation policy was adopted; the Native Commissioner, Belingwe, described how he applied to a sick girl 'castor oil, mustard plaster and later brandy and pneumonia mixture' with 'remarkable results'. In Hartley, the Native Commissioner followed the example of the proprietor of the Shepherds Reef Mine and dosed as many Africans as possible with paraffin and sugar.[15] Mr Edgar, a farmer in Shamva, made use of a cave on his land 'as a quarantine hospital for his African labourers. Each man was given, daily, one tot lamp paraffin and one tot 'dop' (brandy) and was fed on good soup.'[16] Father R. H. Baker at Penhalonga distributed government supplies of 'pneumonia mixture, brandy and mustard', and wrote of the mission's amateur medical efforts with a somewhat gruesome relish:

> [The pupils] really enjoyed the job of making mustard plasters. Another great joke was taking the temperature of the old women who had never before seen a clinical thermometer. . . But the supreme delight of all was to give the children a dose of castor oil.[17]

Some whites at first boasted of the success of these remedies but in the end almost all recognised that Africans believed them to have failed completely. Several Native Commissioners noted that the death rate where European medicine was most freely available – in the towns and mines – was much higher than in the remote rural areas where it was not. The Native Commissioner, Chibi, reported that 'natives have at times been apathetic about taking medicines especially in the lower part of the district where an idea had got about that the high morality at the mines, in the northern part of the district, had been partly caused by natives taking medicine'.[18] In Makoni 'the natives preferred the disease to the remedies'.[19] In Mrewa 'many of them when they heard anyone was near administering medicine ran away and hid . . . They had heard from natives who ran away from Salisbury what was being done there, and they were afraid the same system would be adopted.'[20] Nor did government doctors win confidence in the rural areas. 'There is a marked antipathy toward the medical man', wrote the Native Commissioner, Lomagundi. 'Kindly and sympathetic handling is required as much for the native as the European. It would be of enormous value if Medical men would learn something of the local language.'[21] The 1918 experience made no converts to western medicine. Indeed in Matabeleland it was lamented that where European doctors and clinics had been making ground, Africans had now 'lost much of their confidence in the efficacy of European medicine'.[22]

The pandemic brought few converts to mission Christianity either. Archdeacon Etheridge, noting the closure of schools and the collapse of church offerings, nevertheless tried to look on the bright side: surely the 'extraordinary amount of kindness' shown by whites to Africans 'must have a good effect in drawing the two races together'. Moreover, while 'missionaries have often to meet a certain amount of unpopularity in their work, never during the course of nineteen years' work have I heard so much appreciation of the work of missionaries as during the past two months'.[23] Yet most of this new appreciation came from other Europeans.

It was all very well for the American Methodists in Manicaland to draw the conclusion from the pandemic that what was needed was intensified mission medical effort:

> Sickness among the people has almost no check. Ignorance and superstition go through the land and dead bodies lie in their wake . . .We need at least four good hospitals and sixteen dispensaries. These are essential to the Christian occupation of this land . . . a demonstration of the value and blessing of Christianity.[24]

But the American Methodist Episcopal Church (AMEC) gave out the same rough and ready 'medicines' with the same negative results. The American Methodists might attack the Roman Catholics for their 'medieval attitude' and its replacement of traditional magic by a 'new kind of magic which [the African] imbibes in the name of the living God',[25] but even the Catholics had no liturgical answer to influenza. In short, both scientifically and spiritually the mission churches failed to meet the challenge of the pandemic. Indeed, the African reminiscences about the period which are now preserved in the American Methodist archives reveal how ill-founded their self-confidence was. Jackson Mundirecke Rugayo, one of the African founding fathers of

Methodism, remembered the last months of 1918 mainly in terms of white lack of faith and fraternity. Rugayo was then kitchen-boy at Old Umtali mission where Reverend James imposed a strict defensive quarantine:

> If a visitor came straight into the house through ignorance of the procedure. . . and the 'tough' master came upon him in there, the intruder would be 'tossed' outside with all the dread that accompanies the sight of a seven-headed monster. But really the monster was the influenza germs. In a scene which Jackson recalls vividly, Mr James was conducting the meeting and seated all by himself about ten yards away from the group who sat closely listening to the Chairman who saw concern for immunity outstrip every other consideration.[26]

Significantly enough the only claim I have come across to a decisive missionary victory during the pandemic comes from a very different missionary tradition. The miner Rees Howells, who had been prominent in the Welsh Pentecostal Revival, had joined the South African General Mission at Rusitu in eastern Manicaland. Howells had been working for such a revival in Manicaland but had been meeting the resistance especially of the male elders, committed as they were to the institution of bride-price:

> God had a way that was most unexpected. It was the time of the great Influenza epidemic . . .The Lord then reminded Mr Howells of how, in the intercession for sick people in the village at home [Wales], he had been led to challenge death a number of times. Would he be able to challenge it again here on a much larger scale?

Typically, the disease first afflicted the mission station itself, though no-one died there. During this time 'the heathen said it was a curse from the ancestral spirits, because of the Christians who had broken the lobola (bride-price)'. But:

> soon it reached the kraals also, and many were dying. In two or three days, a deputation came up from the chief and asked 'Have you any deaths?' 'No', replied Mr Howells, 'Have you had any?' 'Yes, many,' they said. 'But can't the witch-doctor do anything to help you?' 'Oh, two of them were among the first to go down.' 'But what about your ancestral spirits?' 'Our fathers never had this illness,' they answered, 'so their spirits cannot deal with it.' 'Quite so', returned Mr Howells. 'The witch-doctors have failed and the ancestral spirits have failed – but our God has not failed.' 'Are none of your people going to die then?' they inquired. The Holy Spirit said to His Servant 'Tell them that no one can die on the station.' So he answered 'No! Not one will die on the mission station.'

There followed a tense few days. Howells invited everyone on to the mission, promising them immunity also, provided that they publicly admitted 'that our God is the living God, and that He can help where the witch-doctors and the ancestral spirits have failed!' So a procession of 'gospel-hardened' men trooped into the mission. Howells found that 'the Holy Spirit was stronger than the 'flu. What it was to live with God in a plague!'

It should be noted that Howells did not rely on the Spirit alone, as later African churches were to do. He made use of his medical skills. 'The Lord gave guidance about the way to do things. He told me to turn the chapel into a hospital and put fires in at night, so that the temperatures were kept even. If I had not had those fifteen months of medical training, I should have been at sea: but there was no need to make a mistake.' Nevertheless, the Rusitu experience during the pandemic was a significant precursor of the rise of the African Spirit Churches.[27]

African explanations of the pandemic

When I first began to think about this topic I made the assumption that the scale and novelty of the influenza pandemic made it almost impossible for Africans to understand it in traditional terms. As the elders said to Howells, 'Our fathers never had this illness so their spirits cannot deal with it.' The first thing I ever read on the subject confirmed me in this view. This was Wulf Sachs' extradordinary psychological biography of John Chavafambira, a migrant and diviner from Manicaland, *Black Anger*. Early in the book Sachs gives us his protagonist's account of the pandemic in eastern Manicaland:

> A terrible disease had fallen upon the land. Kraal after kraal was invaded by the pestilence. People died like flies, and their bodies were hurriedly buried outside the kraal, Christian and pagan alike. There was no time for ritual . . . [None of] the *ngangas* [traditional healers] could do anything. They told the people that the disease came from the white folk. It was not sent by the *midzimu* [ancestors], or by the Mwari [high god], but by the white people. So many were killed in the great war of the white people that the blood of the dead had caused this great sickness.[28]

Such a view, however, underestimates the resilience of existing categories of explanation. Just as many whites were able to persuade themselves that their rough and ready medicines were effective, so many Africans were able to convince themselves that the pandemic was comprehensible and controlled by traditional means. The pandemic, after all, though devastating was very short-lived, all over in a mere two months. It was easy enough to credit one or other agency with having driven the disease away.

Sometimes it was believed that Africans had saved themselves through recourse to their own, more effective, medicines. Thus in an interview with the National Archives Oral Historian, old Sergeant Masotsha Ndlovu, the radical trade unionist and nationalist politician who lies buried in Heroes' Acre in Harare, recalled his days as a migrant worker on Killarney Mine in Filabusi district. Influenza came to the mine in October 1918. 'People would have a headache, cough and they would die. I left Killarney because of that. What saved me is that when I arrived at home [Fort Rixon] people had discovered a certain herb, Ukhalimela, that cured the disease. That is what saved us from death.'[29]

Others sought to deal with influenza in the idiom of witchcraft belief. The pandemic may have affected people of all races, all over the world, but its incidence in the Rhodesian countryside was very uneven, with some homesteads devastated and others nearby unaffected. The Native Commissioner, Chibi, reported that local Africans believed that 'many of the deaths have been caused by unnatural means especially those of families who have lost several of their number while others living in the kraal have lost only a few or none at all'.[30] In early 1919 Native Commissioners' courts throughout the country were full of witchcraft cases. I have been through those for Makoni district, one of which admirably illustrates the co-existence of different ideas of contagion and infection and the way in which an individual death could be interpreted in terms of pre-existing hostilities. In this case the death was that of an unpopular headman's son, Mujenga. Mujenga was on tour in October 1918 collecting tax and moving from kraal to kraal. He passed through Chikundu's kraal, where there were people sick with influenza, and arrived at Nyatzanza's kraal where no-one was ill. He found a beer-drink in progress there, designed to mobilise labour for clearing and planting. Mujenga's arrival at the beer party was not popular – 'some present were rather vexed. They asked him why he moved about at that time and whether he wished to carry infection everywhere', and others were angry because he refused to work in exchange for the beer. 'All drank from the same ladle.' When Mujenga subsequently fell ill and died he told his family that 'he knew the beer had killed him' and that he had been poisoned by the hatred of the organiser of the beer-party, Chakatida. They thereupon accused Chakatida of being a wizard by throwing ashes at his door. For his part Chakatida insisted that the death was due to influenza – and there was much debate at the subsequent court hearing as to whether the symptoms had been those of influenza or wizardry.[31]

This and many other cases show the ambiguity of a witchcraft explanation. Nevertheless, in the aftermath of the pandemic there were demands from African headmen and elders for the restoration of witch-finding and the ordeal. In Hartley district a group of headmen asked 'that the Government should allow the Natives to employ their own doctors for the purpose of finding out the evil-doers among them who are responsible for the sickness . . . which is increasing among the people'. They assured the Native Commissioner that no-one would be killed. 'In the old days . . . we did not kill all those who had been smelt out, we drove them away to the mountain, Domboshawa, and left them there to practice their wicked arts upon one another.'[32]

But this notion of 'moral isolation' was by no means the only traditional metaphysical response to the pandemic. The western and southern areas of Rhodesia were remarkable for the influence of an oracular cult of the High God, Mlimo or Mwari, whose emissaries were sent out from cave shrines. The cult asserted control over the land and its use. People had often appealed to the cult for protection against locusts or animal diseases. Such disasters had equally often been explained by cult authorities as due to past neglect of the observations due to the High God. In such circumstances orders were given that sacrifices and offerings be made to Mlimo/Mwari and that believers observed certain symbolic commandments and taboos. In October 1918 this pattern of injunction and observance was once again repeated. 'The Mlimo or Mwari people have taken advantage of the epidemic to tell the natives to propitiate the Mlimo spirit with black goats', wrote the Native Commissioner, Chibi. 'Natives are killing black goats to propitiate the Mwari and the custom is to wear pumpkin seeds round the neck threaded on "Nokwe" grass as a preventative.'[33] Evidently the swift cessation of the disease confirmed belief in the efficacy of Mwari's forging protection. In 1919 there was what Dr E. P. Makambe has called 'an outburst of traditional religious fervour' finding expression in 'widespread thanksgiving festivities'. 'It is the wish of the Mlimo', wrote Chief Native Commissioner Taylor about such festivities in the Fort Victoria region, 'that the people should show their gratitude for their delivery from the influenza scourge by indulging in wild orgies of beer-bibbing'.[34]

Migrants from Northern Rhodesia, Nyasaland and Mozambique, who made up the great majority of workers on the mines – and many of whom fled into the countryside in October 1918 – could less easily understand the pandemic in terms of this indigenous territorial cult. The established traditional religious idiom appropriate to them was rather the cult of possession by a-social spirits of pestilence. Such a cult sprang up in October 1918 around the mining centre of Selukwe:

> The natives give two causes for the disease. (1) the Europeans. (2) the Foreign Spirit Jukuu. Those who took the first view usually refused to accept help from Europeans – while the others moved with everything they possessed into the bush – made and drank large quantities of beer and wore coloured handkerchiefs – all this to propitiate Jukuu . . . It was said that unless those who had committed sins (such as intercourse with your neighbour's wife, witchcraft etc) proclaimed their acts aloud, they would not recover.[35]

It can be seen, then, that many established African notions and practices proved capable of responding to the pandemic. Nevertheless, the sense of the implausibility of these local idioms to the universality of the influenza certainly *did* exist for many Africans, and was heightened by the subsequent return of severe bouts of 'flu in subsequent years. Such Africans felt that a new spiritual idiom must be developed, superior to and dismissive of both western and traditional medicine and cosmologies of affliction.

The emergence of African spiritual churches

I have quoted above from Arthur Shearly Cripps' *Africans All* to illustrate the melodramatic horror of the pandemic on the mining compounds. In Cripps' little novel this scene is the backdrop for his real story which concerns the rise of African Christian healing. His hero is the prophet Mufambi, whose commission to heal comes to him in the midst of the pandemic. Mufambi goes to the mine where his brother is dying: 'The morning after I reached my brother, I remember rising up just before the sun rose, and standing among the huts and quarters where many sick men lay, and also many dead men. All of a sudden the wind came blowing to me, and I smelled the smell of death.' Mufambi fails to rescue his brother and has to surrender him to the death cart. At this moment of despair he encounters two pupils from a mission school who tell him 'of Jesus, who went about the land casting out devils from the hearts of men . . . how he sent his own friendly spirit to possess us even as unfriendly spirits possess people'. Inspired, Mufambi opens himself to the Holy Spirit and becomes prophet, teacher and healer. He preaches that: 'Jesus was going about Africa day by day now and night by night as an African, since His Spirit, whose name was Munyaradzi, or Comforter, had gained possession of Africans.'[36]

At the time Cripps wrote he was being prophetic himself rather than descriptive since African churches of the spirit had not yet arisen in Southern Rhodesia. Nevertheless, his grasp of the connection between the pandemic and pentecostal inspiration was exact. It was a connection being made all over Africa. John Peel has shown that the Aladura churches of Nigeria arose out of the 'indelible memory' of the pandemic, which left 250,000 dead in southern Nigeria and made Lagos 'a veritable city of the dead'.[37] Bengt Sundkler has shown how Zulu Zionists took the pandemic as 'a terrible sign of the approaching doom . . . a giant cosmic event', and how recovery from influenza was interpreted as prophetic death and rebirth.[38] It was in the midst of the pandemic in lower Zaire, 'when thousands were dying without medical relief', that Simon Kimbangu received his first prophetic call, a voice saying 'I am Christ, I have chosen you.'[39] To this day the Kimbanguist church remembers that in 1918 'in all Kongo there remained no village and no house without a corpse. A little more and the black race would have entirely disappeared.' Kimbangu came as a rescuer.[40] The Nigerian Brotherhood of the Cross and Star describes 1918 as 'the year when the Holy Spirit came into the world'.[41]

Southern Rhodesian African spirit churches arose out of a similar nexus of ideas and claimed a similar pedigree. The pandemic made an impression on the Zimbabwean Christian imagination in all sorts of ways. There was for instance the Manyika Catholic mystic, Patrick Kwesha, who aspired to found his own black missionary order within the church, and who regarded the influenza of 1918 as a blessed chastisement from God: 'From that time onwards I never really got well. The disease grew and grew until it has almost taken me. But I am glad to say, Praised Be God, because after I got the disease I got many great blessings, blessings that if I had not been humbled by this illness I might not have been given.'[42]

In Kwesha's eyes God had sent the influenza to him to see whether his chosen one could bear affliction as patiently as Job. But many Africans in Southern Rhodesia were not ready to bear affliction patiently. They looked to a God who could bring immediate relief from suffering to *His* chosen. This was the God preached by the Pentecostals. We can trace the rise of a pentecostal religious culture in eastern Zimbabwe, where the great black spirit churches were eventually to arise in the early 1930s. In Manicaland, as in southern Nigeria, 1918 was widely thought of as the year when the Holy Spirit came into the world. It was the year, after all, of the great pentecostal revival among the African preachers and teachers of the American Methodist Episcopal

Church. In Manicaland the pandemic had broken into a great wave of healing and miracle as the inspired AMEC evangelists carried their message through the province. Native Department reports show that immediately before the influenza outbreak there was an atmosphere of intense religious expectation. The Superintendent of Natives, Umtali, asserted at the end of September 1918 that American Methodist catechists were 'preaching the second coming and the natives are wildly excited'; the young men were claiming to have communicated with the dead. From neighbouring Mrewa there came on October 11th the complaint of headmen Mrewa himself: 'He does not object to people being taught to read and write . . . but he objected to the "word of God" which drove his people mad.'[43]

The Native Department believed that the coming of the pandemic had put a terrible stop to revivalist enthusiasm, but in the memories of African Christians in eastern Rhodesia the two events became inseparably intertwined. In the years that followed, moreover, Apostolic Faith missionaries from South Africa carried the pentecostal promises to all the Reserves of Manicaland. This was the context for the emergence of the two great Shona *Vapostori*, or Apostolic, churches of Johana Maranke and Johana Masowe in the early 1930s. Their churches were to become international in appeal and to embrace hundreds of thousands of members. Their founders were revered as prophets, entrusted by God with the revelation of a way of living and a way of healing superior either to tradition or to western teaching. Both men forbade the use of medicines of any kind – a prohibition which their followers seek to observe in Zimbabwe today. Both had grown up in the American Methodist strongholds of Manicaland and knew of the combination of pentecost and pandemic in 1918; both had interacted with Apostolic Faith preachers. And both traced back their own ministries to the influenza outbreak.

Johana Maranke, born in 1912, claimed to have commenced his visions of 'the many people he saw on a cloud in the east' in his sixth year, in 1918. As for Johana Masowe – John of the Wilderness – the testimony of one of his acolytes, James Gore, vividly makes all the connections – influenza, the coming of the prophet, the end of the old spiritual order:

> In the year when the influenza was rampant in the country I became ill and remained so for three months. My father used to carry me to Svongosve [a spirit medium] who had a healing spirit. They used some snuff and medicine to cure me . . . At midnight there was a roar of thunder from the east to the west . . . Then the spirit that was in Svongosve spoke

out and said that it was the word of God which had caused this noise. The spirit said that the word of God had fallen somewhere in the east. . . [Then] in 1931 the spirit of Svongosve said 'The child whom I referred to is now grown up' . . . The spirit knew that the time for their departure had come. They said 'We the spirits are going away. The word of God whom you pray to is here. This word of God . . . forbids the use of medicine' . . . Then in 1932 we heard that Baba Johan had come.[44]

Conclusion

In the end, then, the main significance of the influenza pandemic in African medical history may have been in the impetus which it gave to the emergence of anti-medicine movements. Of course, such movements could have emerged – and in parts of Africa already had emerged – without the influenza crisis. Counter-establishment anti-medicine movements were an aspect, after all, of world Christianity in the late nineteenth and early twentieth centuries, whose influence was bound to reach Africa. Moreover, as this chapter has shown, the influenza pandemic did not discredit existing systems of healing and explanation in everyone's eyes. Nevertheless, the pandemic of 1918 with its atmosphere of crisis and with the effective failure of all medical treatment, powerfully assisted and legitimated the emergence of African anti-medicine.

Notes

1 C. A. Mimms, 'The pathogenesis of influenza', in P. Selby (ed.), *Influenza: Virus, Vaccines, Strategy*, Sandoz Institute, Switzerland, 1976, pp. 95-6.

2 I. D. Mills, 'The 1918-19 influenza pandemic: the Indian experience', *Indian Economic and Social History Review*, XXII, 1986, pp. 1-40; K. D. Patterson, 'The influenza epidemic of 1918–1919 in the Gold Coast', *Journal of African History*, 24, 1983, pp. 485-502.

3 I. Phimister, 'The "Spanish" influenza pandemic of 1918 and its impact on the Southern Rhodesian mining industry', *Central African Journal of Medicine*, XIX, 1973, pp. 143-8.

4 L. Brider, 'Lessons of the 1918 influenza epidemic in Auckland', *New Zealand Journal of History*, 16, 1982, pp. 97-121.

5 H. Phillips, 'Black October: the impact of the Spanish influenza epidemic of 1918 on South Africa', doctoral thesis, Cape Town, 1984. Chapter 7 of the thesis is entitled 'What was Spanish 'flu? Medical and lay opinion as to its nature and treatment', and Chapter 8 'Why did it happen? Popular and religious explanations'. Luke Williams is studying at the African Research Institute at La Trobe for a thesis on the historical impact of the 1918 pandemic on Nigeria. See Zvidzai Ndava, 'A study of the 1918–19 Spanish influenza pandemic in Southern Rhodesia (Zimbabwe)', University of Zimbabwe, History Honours Dissertation, 1987, contains some interesting oral interview material on African responses.

6 Taylor's warning is cited in E. P. Makambe, 'The African immigrant factor in Southern Rhodesia, 1890–1930', doctoral thesis, York, 1979, p. 540. Many Native

Commissioners took comfort from the fact that Africans could see whites also dying of the disease and hoped that this would persuade them that it was not a European conspiracy. 'Had the plague affected the natives only', wrote N. S. Taberer, the Superintendent of Natives, Salisbury, 'it is difficult to say what the moral effect would have been amongst them. As it so happened that it affected Europeans and natives alike, and they saw it was a disease that attacked all and sundry, they accepted the inevitable in a calm manner'. Annual Report, S/N, Salisbury, 1918, N 9/1/21, National Archives, Harare.

7 Monthly Report, Chilimanzi, October 1918, N 9/4/35, 2, National Archives, Harare.

8 A. S. Cripps, *Africans All*, London, 1928, pp. 9-10. Cripps worked the testimonies he collected up into a short novel so that the memories cited are expressed in Cripps' notion of an African style.

9 Letter from R. H. Baker, Penhalonga, 2 February 1919, *Southern Rhodesia Quarterly Papers*, CVII, May 1919, pp. 7-11.

10 Review of District Annual Reports, 1918, S/N Bulawayo and Gwelo, N 9/1/21, National Archives, Harare.

11 I am drawing here, with Stephen Thornton's permission, on his unfortunately uncompleted doctoral dissertation draft on the experience of the African population of Bulawayo, and especially on a section of it entitled 'African health care and medicine as a means of control'. All the citations in this passage come from the Town Clerk's correspondence files to which Thornton had access.

12 Review of District Annual Reports, 1918, S/N Bulawayo and Gwelo, N 9/1/21, National Archives, Harare.

13 Monthly Report, Makoni, November 1918, NUA 6/2/8, National Archives, Harare.

14 Annual Report, Belingwe, N 9/1/21.

15 Annual Reports, Inyanga, Melsetter, Belingwe, Hartley, 1918, N 9/1/21.

16 E. A. Logan, 'The Shamva story', *Heritage*, 5, 1985, p. 27.

17 Letter from R. H. Baker, Penhalonga, 2 February 1919, *Southern Rhodesia Quarterly Papers*, CVII, May 1919, pp. 7-11.

18 Annual Report, Chibi, 1918, N 9/1/21

19 Monthly Report, Makoni, November 1918, NUA 6/2/8.

20 Annual Report, Mrewa, 1918, N 9/1/21.

21 Annual Report, Lomagundi, 1918, N 9/1/21.

22 Annual Report, Bulawayo, N 9/1/21.

23 E. H. Etheridge, 'Letters from the Archdeacon of Mashonaland', 14 December 1918, *Southern Rhodesia Quarterly Papers*, CVII, February 1919, pp. 4-5.

24 Report of J. R. Gates, *Official Journal of the Rhodesia Missionary Conference of the American Methodist Episcopal Church*, 1919, p. 33.

25 Report of H. N. Howard, *Official Journal*, 1919, p. 45.

26 'The life of Jackson Mundirecke Rugayo', Muchuma files, Old Umtali Archives.

27 Norman Gruber, *Rees Howells, Intercessor: The Welsh Coal Miner a Prince With God*, Fort Washington, 1952, pp. 178-82.

28 Wulf Sachs, *Black Anger*, Westport, 1972, pp. 31-2. Howard Phillips cites this same passage in his thesis on the pandemic in South Africa and sees parallels with Afrikaner prophetic millenarianism.

29 Interview with Sergeant Masotsha Ndlovu, 8 October 1981, AOH/1, National Archives, Harare.

30 Annual Report, Chibi, 1918, N 9/1/21.

31 Rex versus Manyora, 13 May 1919; Rex versus Ckikundu and Mukwewe, 19 May 1919, Rusape, D 3/33/3, National Archives, Harare. John Iliffe describes a similar response in the Tukuyu district of Tanganyika, where casualties from influenza were particularly heavy and where 'the district officer tried fifteen witchcraft cases attributed to the epidemic and noted that headmen were again administering *mwavi*', the poison ordeal. John Iliffe, *A Modern History of Tanganyika*, Cambridge, 1979, p. 270.

32 Acting Native Commissioner, Hartley to S/N/Salisbury, 9 April 1920, N 3/33/12, National Archives, Harare.

33 Annual Report, Chibi, N 9/1/21; Monthly Report, Chibi, October 1918, N 9/4/35, 2.
34 E. P. Makambe, 'The African immigrant factor in Southern Rhodesia', p. 540.
35 Annual Report, Selukwe, 1981, N 9/1/21.
36 A. S. Cripps, *Africans All*, pp. 30-1.
37 J. D. Y. Peel, *Aladura*, Oxford, 1968, pp. 60-2.
38 B. Sundkler, *Zulu Zion*, London, 1976, pp. 120-5.
39 M. L. Martin, *Kimbangu*, Oxford, 1975, p. 44.
40 W. MacGaffey and J. Janzen (eds.), *An Anthology of Kongo Religion*, Kansas, 1974, p. 131.
41 I owe this information to Dr Gabriel Amadi.
42 Notebook of Patrick Kwesha, containing spiritual reflections and dedicated to an imitation of the life of Christ, in possession of Augustine Kwesha, St. Xavier's, Manyika communal land, translated from the Shona by Emilia Chiteka.
43 S/N/Umtali to Native Commissioner, Mrewa, 27 September 1918; Native Commissioner, Mrewa to S/N/Salisbury, 11 October 1918, N 3/5/1/5, National Archives, Harare.
44 Gore's testimony is cited in C. M. Dillon-Malone, *The Korsten Basketmakers: A Study of the Masowe Apostles*, Manchester, 1978, p. 143. Dillon-Malone dates the 'year when influenza was rampant in the country' to 1928. It is true that a form of influenza was widespread in Southern Rhodesia in 1928, when it was said to have caused 'severe suffering' in Manicaland. (Monthly reports, 1928, S 235.522, National Archives, Harare). There had been other outbreaks in 1919, 1923, 1926 and 1927. More work needs to be done on the subsequent history of influenza. Meanwhile, I think it unlikely that a 'child' heralded in 1928 could have 'grown up' by 1931, so that it may be that Gore was indeed referring to the 1918 epidemic.

CHAPTER NINE

Bilharzia: a problem of 'Native Health', 1900–1950

John Farley

The coincidence of the 'age of imperialism' with the rise of the modern germ theory of disease and the ensuing discoveries in the nature of many tropical diseases, has often led to an assumption that imperialism, whatever its other faults, at least led to an improvement in the health of the indigenous populations. But the tropical or colonial medicine that began in the late 1890s with the founding of the London and Liverpool Schools of Tropical Medicine, grew out of a recognition that the lives of European district officers, missionaries, and military personnel could be preserved more effectively by medical officers with some pre-service training in the diagnosis and treatment of tropical diseases. Thus, although references were continually made to 'the welfare and progress of the races we govern', government policy was concerned primarily with the welfare of white officials.[1] 'You send out soldiers and sailors,' Joseph Chamberlain was quoted as saying, 'and you think you are bound to send medical men to look after them. Do you think of the large staff of able civil servants you send out, and what is being done for them in the event of failing health?'[2] Colonial medicine existed primarily to make the tropics fit for the white man to inhabit. Nevertheless, the benefits and triumphs of tropical medicine have often been counted among the gifts of colonialism; a justification for Britain's and also of America's imperial past.[3]

Bilharzia or schistosomiasis provides a test case by which this claim can be evaluated.[4] Unlike malaria, it was almost exclusively a 'native disease' rarely touching the lives of colonial administrators. An immunological disease induced by eggs of schistosome flukes that live in the blood vessels of the human gut or bladder wall, bilharzia was and is a disease of rural poverty, endemic to most tropical areas except India.[5] It is contracted by exposing the skin to fresh water containing schistosome larvae, called cercariae. These cercariae develop from sac-like bodies or sporocysts in the tissues of fresh-water snails, emerge daily in large numbers, and infect humans by boring through the skin. By examining the motives behind British, American and South African interest in this disease, rather than in diseases that threatened the health of their own officials and kinfolk, one can gain a better understanding of the impact of colonial medicine on 'native health'.

Egypt (1914)

British interest in bilharzia was first stimulated, immediately prior to the First World War, by the belief that the disease constituted a serious threat to their garrison in Egypt. No other people on earth suffer the ravages of bilbarzia to the extent of the Egyptian *Fellaheen*. The figures are astonishing: forty-seven per cent of the entire Egyptian population according to J. Allen Scott's estimate of 1937; sixteen to twenty million in the opinion of two Egyptian workers of the 1970s; eighty per cent of Luxor primary school children from a very recent survey.[6]

Europeans first learnt of the disease in the mid-nineteenth century, when, as part of a series of European-style reforms, attempts were made to improve the quality of medical education in Egypt by hiring European faculty for the medical school in Cairo.[7] One such faculty member, Theodor Bilharz, first described the schistosome worm in 1851, while at the same time another, Wilhelm Griesinger, gave an account of the disease pathology.[8] In the 1890s, a series of similar reforms by the British, who had taken control of the country in 1882, brought Arthur Looss from the University of Leipzig to the faculty. Looss eventually postulated an erroneous life-cycle for the schistosome worm that led the British to take an official interest in bilharzia.

When Looss arrived in Egypt, nothing new had been added to the original observation of Bilharz: the egg hatched to release a 'free embryo' or miracidium, a small free-swimming larval stage that remained viable for only a few hours. What happened next remained a mystery, although many concluded, by analogy with better known parasites, that the miracidium must penetrate the tissues of a snail or other invertebrate intermediate host. But the most authentic statement was to come from Looss, who had rapidly established himself as one of the world's leading helminthologists.

Early in his career in Egypt, Looss naturally assumed that the miracidium most likely developed in a mollusc intermediate host. But failure to experimentally infect snails and bivalves of the Nile Delta, or to find snails and other invertebrates naturally infected with the schistosome larvae led him to conclude, 'that the transfer of the embryo cannot take place by means of an intermediate host from the lower animals'. Thus, according to Looss, the miracidium of schistosomes, after hatching from the egg, does not pass into a snail but penetrates directly back into man. In schistosomes, he argued, the sporocyst larval stages develop in the liver of man, not the digestive gland of snails. 'I am thus forced to the conviction,' Looss wrote, 'that man himself acts as an intermediary host.'[9]

The well-deserved reputation of Looss was such that this bizarre 'skin infection theory' gained widespread support. As Frank Madden, Professor of Surgery at the Egyptian Medical School, noted in the first text devoted exclusively to bilharzia: 'Any small puddle may become defiled with the urine or faeces of a patient suffering from bilharziosis; and, in a very short time, the water or mud is alive with miracidia, which may become applied to the bare feet, legs, or hands, penetrate the skin, and so lead to infection.'[10]

The implications of such a life-cycle are not hard to imagine: a parasite passed directly from man to man in this way would be as potentially dangerous to the white man as to the Egyptian peasant. But it would be particularly threatening to British troops stationed in Egypt and along the Suez canal. Every puddle in every army camp would be a potential source of the disease. Artillery men, returning home from Egypt, could be responsible for an epidemic of bilharzia in Woolwich barracks! The Looss theory of direct transmission had potentially transformed bilharzia into a white man's disease.

The British were not long in responding to this threat. On 24 October 1913, at a meeting of the Advisory Committee of the Tropical Disease Research Fund, Ronald Ross proposed that Dr Stephens of the Liverpool School be sent to Cyprus to investigate the disease. The disease was, he noted, a matter of great importance to Egypt, 'including the British garrison'. The committee decided instead, however, to send Robert Leiper to China, 'to study the mode of spread of bilharziasis and to obtain, if possible, definite experimental evidence on this subject'.[11] The Chinese aspect of the trip was a failure, but a visit to Japan, where the life-cycle of *S.japonicum* had recently been discovered, convinced him that 'the life-cycle of *Schistosoma japonicum* conforms in essential respects with those of other trematodes'.[12] It was similar in that the schistosome miracidium, hatching from the egg, invaded the tissues of snails to produce sac-like sporocysts. In turn these produce a multitude of forked-tailed cercariae that bored into the skin of Japanese workers in the paddy fields. Thus, Leiper concluded in his report to the committee, 'the Looss hypothesis is entirely erroneous. It remains now to be demonstrated that *Schistosoma haematobium* follows a similar course.'

By this time, with Britain at war and poor Looss unceremoniously expelled back to Germany, the solution to the bilharzia riddle in Egypt had become of vital importance to the British garrison. As a result, Leiper was co-opted to the Royal Army Medical Corps and sent out to investigate the disease. His mission was clear:

> In view of the widespread occurrence of an allied disease in Egypt and of the probable employment of large numbers of troops upon the canal defences, I was authorized to proceed to Egypt to investigate bilharzia disease in that country and to advise as to the preventive measures to be adopted in connection with the troops.[13]

Leiper began his investigations by collecting over 3000 snails from a canal at El Marg, a small delta village northeast of Cairo. He soon found the forked-tailed cercariae he had learned to recognise in Japan in two common snail species, and carried back with him to London four mice, twenty-six rats, sixteen desert rats, two guinea pigs and four monkeys experimentally infected wth these cercariae. When examined, all carried schistosome worms in their portal systems. Thus, as in Japan, the life cycle of the Egyptian schistosomes involved passage through snail intermediate hosts and direct penetration of the cercariae into the final host. Looss had been totally wrong.

The practical implications of these findings to the British troops in Egypt were made very clear in Leiper's report. According to the Looss hypothesis, Leiper wrote, 'all transient collections of water are dangerous if freshly contaminated. . . Infected troops would be liable to reinfect themselves, to spread the disease among other troops, and to convey the disease to any part of the world.' On the other hand, 'large bodies of water, such as the Nile, canals, marshes, and birkets, are little liable to be infective'. But now, with discovery of snail hosts, Leiper continued, 'transient collections of water are quite safe . . . Infected troops cannot reinfect themselves or spread the disease directly to others . . . and all permanent collections of water, such as the Nile, canals . . . are potentially dangerous, depending on the presence of the essential intermediary host.'[14]

With these discoveries, Leiper concluded, bilharzia was no longer a threat to a well-disciplined body of troops where regulations to avoid snail-contaminated water could be rigorously enforced. 'We may foretell with reasonable safety,' noted an article in the *Journal of the Royal Army Medical Corps*, 'that the disease will never attain the terrible hold and produce the serious ravages which occur in heavily infected natives of Egypt.'[15] The disease had become, 'one of those diseases for which the individual is mainly, if not entirely, personally responsible'. Bilharzia no longer constituted a serious threat to the well-being of disciplined British troops or to colonial officials living in the approved style. Londoners would not be stricken down by the disease as it moved irresistibly from puddle to puddle across the city. The disease could safely be ignored. In 1939, one year before a new era opened on the medical history of the British Empire, Harold Scott of the London School of Hygiene and Tropical Medicine published his two volume *A History of Tropical Medicine*. No mention was made of bilharzia!

South Africa and Southern Rhodesia

This indifference to bilharzia was not shared by white South Africans, then, of course, still part of the British Empire. By the 1920s they had become very conscious of a new menace to their well-being: 'diseased natives'. Annie Porter, hired by the South African Institute of Medical Research to investigate the occurrence of schistosomes and other helminths in the African population, warned of the danger in her first report. The African, she noted, 'becomes a potentially dangerous nuisance to non-immune hosts, and a disseminating centre for a number of gastro-intestinal troubles as a result of his promiscuous habits'. White children, she warned, were particularly liable to infection by parasites passed to them by their African nurses. Indeed, she concluded, 'it seems very probable that infected natives serve as reservoirs of disease'.[16] C. T. Loram, chairman of a South African committee set up to investigate the possibilities of training natives in medicine, took up the cry. 'There are hordes of natives in many centres,' the report noted, 'who have little chance of medical treatment and the untreated sick become a menace to the rest of the community.'[17] The threat came not so much from specific diseases, but from the 'disease-ridden natives' who carried these afflictions.

But this threat to their own health was not the only factor in encouraging the white community to consider the health of the African population; economic interests were equally important. 'The health of the Bantu mineworker became almost an obsession with the mining companies', wrote Cartwright in his eulogistic column on South African mine doctors, written in 1971 to commemorate the fiftieth anniversary of the Medical Mine Officers Association of South Africa.[18] Like the United Fruit Company and other American companies involved in tropical trade, the mine companies of South Africa eventually built modern hospitals, hired full-time medical staff, and did much to reduce the disease mortality in the mines that had reached horrendous levels after the Chamber of Mines began recruiting unskilled African mine-workers. Also, like their American counterparts, they took an interest in promoting research into tropical diseases and to this end helped to found the South African Institute of Medical Research.[19]

When the mines were reopened, after the Boer War, the Chamber of Mines faced a critical labour shortage. The possibility of bettering the health conditions of the 'mine boys' in order to 'encourage' more recruits, led them to finance a series of health reports. The report of 1903 showed an annual mortality rate of 57.7 per thousand, 41.7 per cent of them from respiratory diseases. Worse again, the report of 1905 showed an almost unbelievable mortality rate of 130 per thousand from Africans recruited from the tropical areas north of the Transvaal border and hand-picked for their physique and good health. That is approximately one-eighth of a work force, consisting entirely of young males, died each year! But it took a decade before the Chamber of Mines began to attack the problem in a serious manner. In 1913 General Gorgas, invited to Johannesburg to advise on sanitation in the compounds of the African mine workers, recommended expanded hospital facilities, more spacious accommodation in the compounds, and a separate bed for each man.[20] A year earlier the mining industry had joined with the Union government to found the South African Insititute for Medical Research, set up to carry out routine bacteriological examinations and to carry out research pertaining specifically to the diseases of African labourers in the gold, diamond and coal mines.

Similar but less dramatic events took place in Southern Rhodesia, where, in 1928, concern for the health of mine workers led to a section entitled 'Native Health' being included in the annual reports of their Health Department. Rhodesians too were apprehensive about their diseased Africans. 'The native is the reservoir,' noted the 1931 report of the Southern Rhodesian Public Health Department, 'from which the white man, who is obliged to live in close contact with him, becomes infected. As instances may be cited, diseases of the type of malaria, dysentery and various intestinal worms, such as Schistosoma.'[21] The realisation that the health of these potentially dangerous Africans had been largely ignored by the medical authorities, galvanized the whites into action. By the mid-1930s, the white settlers in Southern Rhodesia had twenty-five 'native' base hospitals in operation. William Blackie, Director of the Public Health Laboratory, best summed up the rationale for this interest in African health. 'It is reasonable to regard this enterprise as an insurance for the protection of the health of the European,' he wrote, 'and as an investment by the nation for the better maintenance of its labour supplies in quality and quantity.'

> I am no sentimental negrophilist . . . But no matter how much we may dislike it, the native will not permit us either to ignore or forget him unless under penalty of extreme peril to ourselves, since, for a great number of diseases which worry us, the native provides the infected reservoir . . . If I can succeed in awakening the public conscience to this regard, I shall feel that I have performed a greater service to the European community than to the native people.[22]

Bilharzia occupied a fairly prominent place among the major diseases of the African threatening the health and profits of the white population in South Africa and Southern Rhodesia. Blackie himself, as an helminthologist from the London School of Hygiene and Tropical Medicine, had arrived in 1927 to survey the Rhodesian population for helminths (parasitic worms). He found bilharzia to be the most serious helminth disease of white school children, and given the threat posed by 'native reservoirs of disease', recommended a massive helminth survey of the native reserves. This survey, carried out in 1930, showed the disease to be 'of primary importance in the colony'; in many districts approximately twenty per cent of the African children carried the schistosome worm.[23]

Although respiratory diseases naturally took research priority in South Africa, Dr G. A. Turner, medical officer of the Witwatersrand Native Labour Association, had early drawn attention to the incidence of bilharzia among the native mine recruits from Mozambique. 'There is probably no disease,' he wrote in 1910, 'which causes the inhabitants of the Province of Mozambique so much distress and anxiety as bilharziosis. Every evil under the sun, amongst others impotency in men and sterility in women, is attributed to it.'[24] Probably as a result of this warning, bilharzia was included among the diseases investigated by staff members of the South African Insititute for Medical Research. Until her resignation in 1931, Annie Porter took charge of this research, publishing her definitive work on the disease in 1938. Although forced into many mistakes by her inability to identify the snail intermediate hosts and to distinguish the human schistosome larval from the larvae of other schistosomes, she was basically correct in describing the distribution of the disease in the Union. Bilharzia was endemic, she noted, in the Transvaal roughly north of the Mafeking-Pretoria line; in Natal; and in the Cape Province, east of the Drakensburg escarpment and north of the Sundays River and Port Elizabeth.[25]

Treatment and control

Curiously, before the Second World War, despite their belief that 'bilharzia-ridden natives' constituted a threat to their health and prosperity, neither the South Africans nor Southern Rhodesians took action against the disease. The authorities in both countries were content with surveys.

Action was possible; by the 1920s two chemicals seemed poised to eradicate bilharzia: antimony tartrate or tartar emetic and copper sulphate. Both chemicals were believed to be killers. The former, when injected into the bloodstream, was thought to kill the adult parasite; the latter, under laboratory conditions killed snails in low dilutions. The role of both chemicals in the possible eradication of the disease had been discovered shortly after Leiper had described the correct life-cycles of the worms in Egypt. Before this discovery, Looss had argued that eradication depended upon education and complete sanitary control for the *Fellaheen* population. But with the discovery of these chemicals and the snail intermediate hosts, the way was open for western medical technology. The disease could be eradicated by killing snails or the adult worms, and the *Fellaheen* could be allowed to continue in his time-hallowed ways. Bilharzia control involved no social action.

A. C. Chandler, who first discovered the molluscicidal activity of copper sulphate while working in the gorgeous Willamette Valley of Oregon, as far away from the problems of Egypt as one could imagine, noted the attractive features of such chemicals. It offered, or so it seemed, a method of combating disease without involving the patient in any way. It appealed to the scientist and to the politician. The former could now deal with dilutions of chemicals rather than trying to understand the way of life of illiterate peasants; the latter could ignore the painful and politically explosive notion of upgrading and changing the lives of the masses, by opting instead for a simple mollusc-killing chemical. 'The fact', Chandler wrote, 'that fluke infections may possibly be controlled by attack upon an intermediate host instead of by reliance upon the enforcement of sanitary regulations makes the ultimate eradication of these infections, in spite of their relative incurability, a matter of brighter prospect than is the case with many other verminous parasites.'[26] But Chandler was wrong in one respect; when he wrote these words bilharzia was no longer regarded as an incurable disease. In 1918 Dr J. B. Christopherson in the Sudan announced that thirty grains of tartar emetic given over a fifteen to thirty day period 'is a definite cure for bilharziasis'.[27]

But initially neither of these chemicals were used in South Africa or Southern Rhodesia against the disease in the African population. Action against bilharzia was taken only when segments of the white population were found infected with the disease. By the mid-1920s, children of poor Boer farmers in the Transvaal had been found with bilharzia, representing the only Europeans in Africa to be seriously threatened by the disease. The response was immediate; beginning in 1927, Afrikaaner schoolchildren were collected together in 'summer camps' at various sites throughout the Transvaal and given the standard intravenous injections of tartar emetic. By 1929 a Transvaal Bilharzia Committee had been formed to oversee the programme and set up educational and publicity programmes. English and Afrikaans signs were posted at swimming holes warning children of the danger in the water. By 1932, with enthusiasm for the treatment camps on decline, the committee decided to press for bilharzia-free swimming pools in the schools of white farm children in which the water could also be used for irrigation. Although, in the Transvaal, a brief and unsuccessful attempt was made to open a similar camp for African children, in Natal, where white farmers were more wealthy than their Transvaal counterparts and bilharzia was limited to the African population, no attempt was made to copy the Transvaal example. Bilharzia would only be attacked if it infected the white population.[28]

If, in the 1920s and 1930s, the South Africans were unwilling to spend money on the chemical treatment and prevention of bilharzia among the black population, they were certainly not prepared to attack the root causes of this and other diseases. But, again, a different set of rules operated for the white community. For the Labour-Nationalist government of General Hertzog, elected in 1924 on a platform of white supremacy and black segregation, the presence of disease-ridden poor whites, their own kith and kin, was a matter of urgent concern. In 1927 the Union government and the Dutch Reform Church requested the assistance of the Carnegie Foundation in an investigation of 'poor whitism'. The Carnegie Commission, reporting in 1932, painted the picture of landless rural 'bywoners', poor settlers with small land holdings, unskilled labourers, and pioneer-type nomads. Usually of Dutch-German extraction, poorly educated if not illiterate, speaking only Afrikaans and weakened by disease, they remained isolated from the mainstream of European progress, psychologically unable to adjust to modern conditions.[29]

Bilharzia, or 'human red-water disease' as it was locally known, was reported to be a major problem among the children of poor whites. 'We have no hesitation whatever in stating', the report noted, 'that, as a school disease, "red-water" ranks but slightly inferior, as far as its debilitating power is concerned, to hookworm disease and malaria.'[30] But the recommended solution to these health problems was not to be insecticides, molluscicides or tartar emetic. 'Poverty and unsatisfactory diet', the report concluded, 'generally had a more detrimental effect than malaria or other diseases.' The economic system, not disease, was the root cause of all other problems. The system created poverty and ignorance among the poor whites, which in turn led to malnutrition, and the weakening of resistance to disease.[31] Even though the children of the poor whites were treated with tartar emetic, the South African government was made aware that the root problems were economic. For the first and only time a government set out to eliminate a bilharzia health problem by economic and social means. But, for the first and only time the patients were white, not black.[32]

The Americans

Before the outbreak of the Second World War, few outside Egypt, South Africa, and Southern Rhodesia, would have listed bilharzia as a major tropical disease. But by the end of the war, the disease had been elevated to number six in the world, and it would rise rapidly thereafter to take up a position immediately behind malaria. This increase in status did not arise because of a general concern with the health of third world countries or because of its general impact on the allied armies in the war. Indeed, with only forty-two cases of the disease reported from British and Commonwealth troops fighting in North Africa and the Middle East, the British medical history of the war dismissed the disease with the casual statement that 'by the application of simple precautionary measures based on knowledge gained during the war of 1914-18, there was no repetition of the outbreak which then occurred in Egypt'.[33] The Australian historians took a similar position. The American Army, on the other hand, reported over 2,500 cases of schistosomiasis, but such a number is miniscule compared with those of malaria and venereal diseases to say nothing of the battle casualties suffered during their bloody war with Japan. But one campaign played a major role in bringing schistosomiasis to the front line of tropical diseases: Leyte 1944.

In August 1944, the Americans decided to pass over the invasion of Mindanao, as previously planned, and to jump directly north to Leyte, an island where the disease is endemic. The landing took place on October 20th, and by Christmas Day the campaign was virtually over. Out of 257,766 men who took part in the operation, the US Army sustained 15,584 casualties with 3,508 killed.[34] In December bilharzia suddenly appeared among American troops admitted to the 118th Field Hospital; 80 cases in December; 155 in January. By the end of that month the hospital adjutant reported,'the situation regarding manpower is becoming critical. Number of cases of schistosomiasis have been diagnosed.'[35] By May 1945 the total number of cases on the island had climbed to over 1,000.

With fear of a full-scale epidemic mounting, a major military operation against schistosomiasis geared into action. An extensive educational programme got underway with posters, cartoons, and mobile demonstration laboratories. In February the 5th Malarial Survey unit and a Medical Research Unit were attached to the 118th Field Hospital to study various aspects of the disease; in April a Sub-commission on Schistosomiasis, appointed by the Army Epidemiological Board in Washington, arrived to study the problem; and a month later a three-man team from the Naval Research Unit arrived on the island with similar goals in mind. The men who manned these various units, F. Bang, N. Hairston, O. Graham, M. Ferguson, E. Faust, W. H. Wright, D. B. McMullen, and G. W. Hunter III were to put schistosomiasis on the academic map of the United States after the war by publishing their war-time findings in the *American Journal of Hygiene* and *American Journal of Tropical Medicine*. These reports appeared at a very auspicious time for the development of career opportunities in tropical medicine in the United States, for by the end of the war members of the tropical medicine community in the United States were desperately seeking ways of preventing a return to the 'bad old days'.

In these wretched days of the 1920s and 1930s, the American Society of Tropical Medicine, after a bright beginning, had degenerated into a rump group of the Southern Medical Association. By the First World War, the Society, founded in 1903, had established itself as a successful, albeit small, professional body that included among its members all the eminent figures in the discipline. But over the next decade, with the flush of empire diminished, the war at an end and finally the Depression, there seemed little interest in the subject and financial support was non-existent. In 1934, in an attempt to counter this disturbing trend, leaders in the field formed the American Academy of Tropical Medicine whose role was not only to educate the American public, further knowledge and be a general source of expertise, but more significantly to receive and administer research funds.[36] They in turn set up the American Foundation of Tropical Medicine specifically to solicit these funds.

Following the 1935 joint meeting of the American Society and American Academy of Tropical Medicine in St Louis, described by one enthusiast as 'one of the great moments in the development of tropical medicine in the United States', the Foundation was officially created. Presided over by Perry Burgess, President of the Wood Memorial (a fund directed at leprosy in the Philippines), and including the Presidents of Johns Hopkins, Columbia and the University of California as well as business executives from the Firestone Rubber Company and the United Fruit Company, the Foundation held their first meeting in April 1936, where they discussed 'a carefully worked out case for tropical medicine'.[37] To solicit the necessary funds, they agreed, it was first necessary to learn from members of the Academy specifically what was needed. But this simple task proved to be a problem. 'The research projects submitted by members of the Academy are, for the most part, entirely too vague', they noted in their first progress report, and 'do not appear to be specific enough to warrant their use for the purpose of raising funds.' In addition, the report continued in its very forthright manner, there were so few research plans submitted 'that perhaps there is not the real need for support of research in tropical medicine among American workers that we have been led to believe there was'.[38] Similar dissatisfaction was expressed in 1939; members of the Foundation wanted to know from the Academy, 'what programme you have in view, what your policy is to be, what your plans are to be, and what the chances are of making the Foundation a going concern'.[39] Clearly tropical medicine in the United States was not enjoying vintage years.

Nevertheless, as the secretary of the Foundation noted in his annual report of that year, 'the time is peculiarly appropriate for a major effort in the field of tropical medicine in the Western Hemisphere'. The stimulus was not the war that had already started in Western Europe, but the 'Good Neighbor' policy of Franklin Roosevelt's New Deal.[40] In 1938, to increase cultural and educational relationships with the other American republics to the south, required by this new policy, the United States formed the division of Cultural Relations. As a result, the secretary recommended that the Foundation devote their activities to aid teaching and research in tropical medicine in these republics. Grants should be given to US medical schools to set up post-graduate courses in tropical medicine similar to those in London, and graduate fellowships should be established for each of the American republics for study in the US.[41] Not surprisingly, the Council of the American Academy of Tropical Medicine unanimously approved the secretary's recommendations and the American Society of Tropical Medicine expressed 'its sympathetic interest in the activity of the American Academy of Tropical Medicine in increasing inter-American co-operation in the fields of tropical medicine and parasitology'.[42] By 1940 eight $1,000 fellowships in tropical medicine had been granted to Latin American nationals for a six month post-graduate course in tropical medicine at Tulane, although two years later the Foundation was financially unable to continue with these scholarships. But by then a new situation had arisen that offered far more scope than poverty-ridden republics to the south: the Americans had entered the Second World War.

'The war has placed our society in a position of real importance', announced Dr Thomas Mackie, President of the American Society of Tropical Medicine, in his presidential address of April 1941, eight months before Pearl Harbour and the German declaration of war. With the war, the status of the discipline rose even higher. Membership in the Society jumped from 546 in 1941, to 674 in 1942, 901 in 1943 and 1,213 in 1944.[43] Members now served on committees of the National Research Council, and the Public Health Department, and most significantly advised the Surgeon-General's Office on control and treatment of tropical diseases to which the US forces could be exposed. In addition, the Division of Cultural Relations had been replaced by the Office of the Co-ordinator of Inter-American Affairs aimed at the cultural and commercial aspects of American defence. Health and sanitation took up such an important place in this policy, that in 1942 a subsidiary corporation, the Institute of Inter-American Affairs, was formed to improve health conditions in strategic areas, and to demonstrate through health 'the tangible benefits of democracy', so as to eliminate 'a fertile field for Nazi propaganda'.[44]

The war had brought money, increased membership and an enhanced status to tropical medicine. But would this state of affairs last; or would these be fleeting blessings to disappear as soon as events returned to normal? Thus, a Committee on War and Post-War Problems was set up as early as 1942 to promote post-war research and education in tropical medicine, and in 1945 the Society forwarded a resolution to President Truman, expressing concern 'lest tropical medicine be allowed to deteriorate to its pre-war level'. Present training and research was 'woefully inadequate', they reminded the President, because of which the US Army and Navy had to establish emergency educational programmes at the beginning of the war. 'We therefore recommend', they concluded, 'immediate and active development of this important phase of American medicine.'[45]

In the 1944 report of the Committee on War and Post-War Problems, seven tropical diseases were listed as being significant to the future: malaria, amoebiasis, filariasis, hookworm, leishmaniasis, schistosomiasis and echinococcosis.[46] This list was of major significance in the schistosomiasis story; for the first time the disease had been counted as one of the major health problems of the world. Then, five months later, the schistosomiasis problem exploded in Leyte. For practitioners of tropical medicine, looking to retain their place in the sun, the Leyte campaign could not have come at a more opportune time.

Academic interest in the disease followed quickly. The Philippine articles appeared between 1946 and 1948 mostly in the *American Journal of Hygiene* published by Johns Hopkins University, while in the same period *The American Journal of Parasitology* started carrying increasing numbers of articles on the disease. In 1947, Norman Stoll, President of the American Society of Parasitology, a society with very strong links with tropical medicine, published his famous paper 'this wormy world', in which he estimated 114 million people to be infected with the three human schistosome species.[47] Bilharzia occupied an important place at the 1950 meeting of the American Society of Tropical Medicine, where its President, W. H. Wright, claimed the disease to be 'the most important tropical disease in the world today'.[48]

To justify spending money on tropical diseases, economic arguments were generally used: before backward areas of the world could be developed in order to bolster world trade and provide markets for the US economy, tropical parasites needed to be eradicated or controlled. With improved health in these areas, W. H. Wright noted in 1950, 'we may expect an improved economy, greater production, and an expanded trade with these countries which are rich in raw materials which this country lacks and acutely needs'.[49] Their endeavours to raise money now met with some success. In 1944, for example, the American Foundation of Tropical Medicine obtained $75,000 for use in teaching and research, $15,000 of which went to Tulane, and the Firestone Rubber Company donated $25,000 for research on trypanosomiasis in Liberia. Members of the Society also emphasised the threat posed by tropical diseases to the United States itself. In particular they warned of the danger of returning troops introducing tropical diseases to the country and of American physicians ill equipped to deal with them. Bilharzia loomed large in these arguments.

'It is not beyond reason', Andrew Warren, chairman of the War and Post-War Committee noted in 1944, 'to expect that *Schistosoma mansoni* cases might have operations for cancer and haemorrhoids, *S. haematobium* cases have kidneys removed'.[50] In 1946 a search for potential snail hosts in North America became a priority item when a few individuals of the snail *Tropicorbis havanensis*, taken from a pond on the campus of Louisiana State University at Baton Rouge, were found to liberate cercariae after exposure to the miracidia of *S.mansoni*.[51]

Conclusion

If the story of bilharzia is typical of other 'native diseases', then the medical policies of the British, British settlers, South Africans and Americans were never much concerned with 'native' health for reasons that did not at the same time serve their own interests. Before the Second World War the diseases of the diseased 'native' would need to threaten or seem to threaten the health or economic prosperity of European troops or settlers before action would be taken. Similarly, after the Second World War, the 'discovery' of bilharzia by the Americans not only reflected an increased interest in tropical diseases stimulated by strategic and trade considerations in tropical America, but also a concern that such diseases constituted a health threat to the United States. But above all, perhaps, the increased interest in tropical diseases after the war stemmed from the activities of academic pressure groups. In the final analysis, the greatest benefactors of this increased activity were American and British research workers; experts to whom the study of tropical diseases provided career opportunities undreamed of in earlier years.[52] The implications are profound: bilharzia has become another westernised disease, to be scientifically researched in the laboratories of North America and Europe, and to be controlled by improved molluscicides and chemical therapy. Meanwhile the very real problems of poverty and malnutrition, with which bilharzia and most other tropical diseases are intimately linked, have become essentially buried.

Notes

This chapter is part of a broad study of the history of tropical medicine in the British and American empires, with special emphasis on bilharzia. I wish to thank the Social Sciences and Humanities Research Council of Canada who have generously supported this work by operating grants and a Leave Fellowship.

1 Quotation from an address by Lord Sheffied at a dinner of the London School of

Tropical Medicine, October 1909, in *London School of Tropical Medicine and Hospital for Tropical Diseases: Miscellanea (1899–1927)*. This publication contains many addresses that discuss both the health of the 'natives' and, in the words of Patrick Manson at the opening of the School on 2 October 1899, the necessity of 'helping our countrymen to carry out some of the duties imposed by the circumstances of race'.

2 Quoted by chairman of the Royal Colonial Institute before an address by Patrick Manson, 'A school of tropical medicine', *Journal of the Royal Colonial Institute*, V, 1900, pp. 309-37.

3 In 1898 the Americans, following their brief war with Spain, took control of Cuba, Puerto Rico and the Philippines and began a series of public health programmes directed against yellow fever, smallpox, cholera, the plague and other diseases. These campaigns, carrried out under the umbrella of American 'tutelage', were seen as one
3 of the great advantages imposed by American civilisation, 'bringing to the Filipinos', for example, 'vivid evidence of the humanitarianism and benevolent intentions of the United States'. J. Gates, *Schoolbooks and Krags: the US Army in the Philippines 1898–1902*, Westport, Conn., 1973. See also Reynaldo Ileto's chapter in this volume.

4 The terminology surrounding the disease is confused. In the mid-nineteenth century, the parasitic worms were placed in a number of different genera, including *Bilharzia*, named to honour Theodor Bilharz, the discoverer of the parasitic worm, and *Schistosoma*. Thus for many years the disease was known as bilharziasis or simply bilharzia (preferred by the British) or schistosomiasis (the American favourite). But in 1954, the International Commission of Zoological Nomenclature recommended that bilharziasis be used to designate the disease. Unfortunately this recommendation has not been followed and today schistosomiasis, or its ugly derivative 'schisto', is generally used.

5 There are three major schistosome species infecting man: *Schistosoma japonicum*, endemic to China, Japan (where it has almost disappeared) and the Philippines: *Schistosoma haematobium*, endemic to the Middle East and virtually the entire African continent; and *Schistosoma mansoni*, endemic to much of Africa and the Middle East, to parts of South America, and some Caribbean Islands including Puerto Rico. For the best account of the disease see Peter Jordan and Gerald Webbe, *Schistosomiasis. Epidemiology, Treatment and Control*, London, 1982.

6 These and other figures can be found in M. F. Abdel-Wahab, *Schistosomiasis in Egypt*, Boca Raton, 1982, p. 7.

7 For details of these reforms see J. Heyworth-Dunne, *An Introduction to the History of Education in Modern Egypt*, London, 1939.

8 An English translation of these papers is incuded in B. H. Kean et al (eds.) *Tropical Medicine and Parasitology*, 2 vols., Ithaca, 1978.

9 A. Looss, 'What is *Schistosomum mansoni* Sambon, 1907?', *Annals of Tropical Medicine and Parasitology*, II, 1908, pp. 153-91; 'The life-history of the bilharzia worm', *Cairo Journal of Science*, IV, 1910, pp. 134-9.

10 Frank Madden, *Bilharziosis*, London, 1907, p. 15.

11 For details of the discussion surrounding this decision see Miscellaneous Papers, Colonial Office, CO 885/22/274.

12 Leiper's report of 15 January 1915 in *Report of the Advisory Committee for the Tropical Disease Research Fund for the year 1914*. Details of the expedition are given in G. S. Nelson, 'A milestone on the road to the discovery of the life-cycles of the human schistosomes', *American Journal of Tropical Medicine and Hygiene*, XXVI, 1977, pp. 1093-1100. A summary of the pioneering Japanese work on the schistosomes, that has never received the honour it is worth, has recently been made available to English readers in M. Sasa, 'An historical review of the early Japanese contributions to the knowledge of *Schistosoma japonica*', in M. Yokagawa (ed.) *Research in Filariasis and Schistosomiasis*, 2, Baltimore, 1972; Kean, *Tropical Medicine and Parasitology*, also contains translations of some of these Japanese papers.

13 Leiper's report to Tropical Disease Research Fund, 21 October 1915, CO 885/23/301.

14 Leiper's 'Report on the results of the bilharzia mission in Egypt, 1915', was published in six parts: *Journal of the Royal Army Medical Corps*, XXV, 1915, pp. 1-55; XXVI 1915, pp. 147-92; XXVI, 1915, pp. 253-67; XXVII, 1916, pp. 171-90; XXX, 1918, pp. 235-53; XXX, 1918, pp. 253-60.

15 A. R. Ferguson, 'Some notes on bilharziasis', *Journal of the Royal Army Medical Corps*, XXIX, 1917, pp. 57-65.

16 A. Porter, 'A survey of the intestinal entozoa both protozoal and helminthic, observed among natives in Johannesburg', *Memoir No.11, South African Institute for Medical Research*, Johannesburg, 1918.

17 *Report of the Committee appointed to Inquire into the Training of Natives in Medicine and Public Health*, Pretoria, 1928, p. 4.

18 A. P. Cartwright, *Doctors of the Mines*, Cape Town, 1971, p. 2.

19 J. F. Murray, 'History of the South African Institute for Medical Research', *South African Medical Journal*, XXXVII, 1963, pp. 389-95.

20 Details from Cartwright, *Doctors of the Mines*.

21 *Southern Rhodesia: Annual Report on Public Health for the Year 1931*, p. 17.

22 *Southern Rhodesia: Annual Report on Public Health for the Year 1936*, pp. 10-11.

23 This work is reported in *Southern Rhodesia: Annual Report on Public Health for the Year 1927, 1928, and 1930.* Also William Blackie, *A Helminthological Survey of Southern Rhodesia*, Memoir Series 5, London School of Hygiene and Tropical Medicine, 1932.

24 G. A. Turner, 'An account of some of the helminthes occurring among South African natives', *Journal of Tropical Medicine and Hygiene*, XIII, 1910, pp. 33-40; 50-9.

25 A. Porter, *The Larval Trematoda found in certain South African Mollusca with special reference to Schistosomiasis (Bilharziasis)*, Johannesburg, 1938.

26 A. C. Chandler, 'Control of fluke diseases by destruction of the intermediate host', *Journal of Agricultural Research*, XX, 1920, pp., 192-208.

27 J. B. Christopherson, 'The successful use of antimony in bilharziosis', *Lancet* II, 7 September 1918, pp. 325-7.

28 Reports of this campaign were given in *Union of South Africa Department of Public Health: Annual Report* for the years after 1927.

29 The report was issued in 5 volumes: Vol.I, J. F. W. Grosskopf, *Economic Report: Rural Impoverishment and Rural Exodus*; Vol.II, R. W. Wilcocks, *Psychological Report: the Poor White*; Vol.III, E. G. Malherbe, *Educational Report: Education and the Poor White*, Vol.IV, W. A. Murray, *Health Report: Health Factors in the Poor White Problem*, Vol.V, J. Albertyne and M. E. Rothmann, *Sociological Report: The Poor White Society and The Mother and Daughter in the Poor Family*. Each of these volumes is self-contained in that the joint findings and recommendations of the entire programme are included.

30 Murray, *Health Report*, pp. 117-19.

31 'Joint findings and recommendations', pp. xiv and xx of each report.

32 The government introduced a series of measures aimed at increasing the prosperity of the 'poor white' Afrikaan community and eliminating the economic threat posed by the equally unskilled African. These included farm credit programmes; improvements in farm marketing; inducements for farm resettlement; and recognition of Afrikaans as an official language, thereby opening up new opportunities for unilingual Afrikaners. These are discussed very briefly in T. H. R. Davenport, *South Africa. A Modern History*, Toronto 1977; and W. Vatcher, *White Laager: The Rise of Afrikaner Nationalism*, London, 1965.

33 J. S. K. Boyd, 'Advances in tropical medicine', in V. Zachery Cope (ed.), *History of the Second World War: Medicine and Pathology*, London, 1952.

34 The Leyte campaign is described in S. E. Morison, *History of the United States Naval Operations in World War II, 12, Leyte, June 1944 – January 1945*, Boston, 1958. For the most detailed account of the schistosomiasis problem in the war, see M. S. Ferguson and F. B. Bang, 'Schistosomiasis', in *Medical Department US Army, Preventive Medicine in World War II*, V, *Communicable Diseases*.

35 Adjutant's Report, Johns Hopkins Hospital 118 in Philippines and Australia, Chesney Archives, Johns Hopkins University Medical School, Baltimore.

36 The fifty-member American Academy of Tropical Medicine, founded in February 1934 with Theobald Smith as President, was open to any US citizen 'who has conducted and published meritorious original investigations' and ' whose scientific interest is, to a definite degree, devoted to one or more problems in this field'. Articles of Incorporation, Archives of the American Society of Tropical Medicine, Countway Library, Harvard University Medical School.

37 'A carefully worked out case for tropical medicine', Directors meeting, American Foundation of Tropical Medicine, 22 April 1936. Archives, American Society of Tropical Medicine.

38 Progress Report to Board Members of the American Foundation and Council Members of the American Academy of Tropical Medicine, 11 November 1937. Archives, American Society of Tropical Medicine.

39 Report of the American Foundation to the 6th Annual Meeting of the American Academy of Tropical Medicine, November 1939. Archives, American Society of Tropical Medicine.

40 This policy marked a change from earlier years when, under the guise of 'tutelary democracy' and 'dollar diplomacy', force was used as a legitimate weapon to protect American business interests. The conventions signed at Montevideo in 1933 and Buenos Aires in 1936 in which the various states 'declare inadmissible the intervention of anyone of them, directly or indirectly, and for whatever reason, in the internal of external affairs of any other of the Parties', represented a change to a policy of 'reciprocity', in which, hopefully, a policy of goodneighbourliness by the Americans would be reciprocated. Bryce Wood, *The Making of the Good Neighbor Policy*, New York, 1961.

41 Secretary's report to the 6th Annual Meeting of the American Academy of Tropical Medicine, Memphis 1939. Archives, American Society of Tropical Medicine.

42 Secretary of American Society to Secretary of American Academy of Tropical Medicine, 31 January 1940. Archives, American Society of Tropical Medicine.

43 Figures from Ernest Faust, 'The American Society of Tropical Medicine. A brief biographical sketch', *American Journal of Tropical Medicine*, XXIV, 1944, pp. 63-9.

44 'Health and Sanitation', in *History of the Office of the Co-ordinator of Inter-American Affairs*, Washington, 1947.

45 Resolution to President Truman, presented at General Meeting of the American Society of Tropical Medicine, December, 1945. Archives, American Society of Tropical Medicine.

46 Schistosomiasis had hardly been noticed by the Society up to that time. In 1906 Stiles presented a paper on *S. japonicum*, Gonzales Martinez had discussed the disease in Puerto Rico at the 1916 meeting, and a paper on *S. mansoni* had been read at the 1932 meeting. An article on *S. japonicum* by Alfred Reed of the Yale Hospital, China appeared in the 1915 volume of *American Journal of Tropical Diseases and Preventive Medicine*, published out of Tulane. In the first volume, published in 1913, a discussion entitled 'is the importance of intestinal parasites in tropical pathology exaggerated?' led Charles Craig to conclude that hookworm was the only worm of any importance, while 'Schistosomum is important, but its locale is limited and the number of cases is small.'

47 Norman Stoll, 'This wormy world', *Journal of Parasitology*, XXXIII, 1947, pp. 1-18.

48 W. H. Wright, 'Medical parasitology in a changing world. What of the future?', *Journal of Parasitology*, XXXVII, 1951, pp. 1-12.

49 *Ibid.*

50 Report of the Committee on War and Post-War Problems, 7 July 1944, presented at General Meeting of the American Society of Tropical Medicine, St Louis, November 1944. Archives, American Society of Tropical Medicine.

51 E. B. Cram and V. S. Files, 'Laboratory studies on the snail host of *S. mansoni*', *Journal of the American Society of Tropical Medicine*, XXVI, 1946, pp. 715-20. H. Stunkard, 'Possible snail hosts of human schistosomiasis in the United States', *Journal of Parasitology*, XXXII, 1946, pp. 539-52. Also a series of articles on the same theme in *Studies on Schistosomiasis*, N. I. H. Bulletin 189, Washington.

52 The study of tropical diseases also provided new careers for British experts after the war. By then the British Colonial Office had become an agent of social and political development for the colonial peoples. A series of Colonial Development and Welfare Acts (1940, 1945, 1950, etc.) allocated over £24 million for research, of which nearly £6.5 million went towards medical research. As in the American case, one can argue that the British were the main benefactors of this activity. The money provided a new career opportunity for British physicians, entomologists and malacologists in the Colonial Research Service.

CHAPTER TEN

The discovery of colonial malnutrition between the wars

Michael Worboys

Introduction

The fact that a large proportion of the world's population is malnourished is common knowledge. Organisations like Oxfam and the Save the Children Fund continually make us aware of the problem and appeal for our help in improving the plight of the 'starving millions' in third world countries. Recent experience, particularly the situation in Ethiopia, suggests that while the consciences of people in rich countries can be pricked by major famines, they remain largely indifferent to the far more pervasive and ultimately more serious problems of undernutrition and malnutrition. There are many reasons why this might be so, but one of the most important seems to be that famines are necessarily short-term crises with definite origins and limits, whereas chronic malnutrition is seen to be a problem that has been and will always be with us. Such views are in fact mistaken. The problem of malnutrition in third world countries, then colonial territories, was first 'discovered' between the wars. Clearly, there had been some awareness of nutritional problems before then, not least with regard to famines, but it was only then that the matter was constructed as an imperial problem and put on the world political agenda. Several questions arise about this particular moment. Why was malnutrition 'discovered' then and not earlier or later? What agencies were responsible for the 'discovery' and how was the problem viewed by different agencies? What approaches and solutions were suggested, formulated and tried?

Although few studies have been made of nutrition in pre-colonial and colonial societies, the three general accounts of the origin of the world food problem all agree that the problem was first recognised between the wars. One view suggests that the peoples of these countries have always had a poor and limited diet due to their low level of subsistence and ignorance of dietetics.[1] Hence, it is claimed that nutritional problems have always been endemic, but that they remain submerged until revealed by the new knowledge of nutrition in the 1930s. A second account is offered by neo-Malthusians who argue that population growth in this century has produced 'too many people' for the available food supply and that this has led to malnutrition becoming the great endemic disease problem of the twentieth century.[2] A third version also claims that the nutritional problems of developing countries are of recent origin, but sees them as deriving from colonialism and especially the destruction of indigenous food production as colonial peoples increasingly switched to producing cash crops for export.[3] By this account malnutrition in developing countries is a true epidemic, an exceptional and widely prevalent crisis of health brought about by special causes not generally present in the affected locality.

Alongside these broader historical perspectives, this topic raises several issues in the historical sociology of medical knowledge. There has, first of all, been singularly little discussion of the diffusion of medical knowledge. Until very recently, medical historians worked with a model that assumed the passive diffusion of a universally valid system of knowledge. However, scholars now recognise the necessity of exploring the mechanisms of the transfer of knowledge and the adaptation and incorporation of that knowledge in different political, cultural and geographical circumstances.[4] Secondly there is an increasing tendency to approach disciplines like nutrition not just as a body of ideas, but as social institutions with contingent affiliations, boundaries and contents.[5] These considerations are particularly germane in the case of nutrition which has many interdisciplinary links both within and between the different natural sciences and social sciences. Finally, and no less critically, there is the way in which medical and scientific knowledge shapes and is used in wider social and political debates. Many writers have argued that this century has seen a growing tendency to 'scientise' or 'medicalise' social problems; that is, moving a problem away from the social domain where something might be done about it and where various political alternatives could be considered, to the natural domain where the problem is treated as immutable or soluble in the 'one right way' defined by experts.[6] In the case of nutrition, 'objective' definitions of poverty levels have led in some cases to the politicisation of individuals and to radical social and political views and programmes. However, approaching the problem of poverty via nutrition has also resulted in the problem being depoliticised. In such instances, remedies are often sought, not through structural changes, but by 'technical fixes'; for example, the supply of dietary supplements and nutritional education.[7]

Discovery

The first official government acknowledgement of nutritional problems in the Colonial Empire in this century came with livestock rather than people! In 1925, heavy stock losses in South Africa and the Kenyan Highlands were serious enough to be referred to a new Cabinet advisory body, the Committee of Civil Research (CCR).[8] The CCR was established to co-ordinate 'economic, scientific and statistical research in relation to civil policy and administration', and it worked by devolving responsibility for particular investigations to expert committees which in turn sought funding and oversaw research work. The response to the stock losses in Africa was typical of the way the CCR worked. A sub-committee on the Mineral Content of Pastures was appointed after informal discussions with relevant experts and by the time of its first meeting, a research proposal had been worked out and the name of the researcher pencilled in.[9] The man chosen to undertake the preliminary survey was John Boyd Orr, then head of the Rowett Research Institute in Aberdeen.[10] The appointment was significant because it launched an influential career in nutritional research and policy, which eventually led to Boyd Orr becoming the first director of the United Nations Food and Agriculture Organisation. He originally qualified in medicine, but after war service he took up work on animal nutrition at Rowett, a new livestock and dairying research establishment concentrating on mineral deficiency conditions. Boyd Orr's career brought together two important trends in post-war British science policy, the new commitment to state-funded applied research and the new interest in nutrition engendered by the discovery of vitamins.[11] Interestingly, Boyd Orr himself was suspicious of many of the claims being made for vitamins and championed minerals as being of equal, if not greater, importance. Scientific and professional interests combined to make him a champion of the British dairy industry and a particular opponent of, what he regarded as, food faddism, especially vegetarianism. He was, between the wars, the main promoter of the provision of daily school milk in British schools. His activities led him to write his famous book, *Health, Income and Nutrition* and to become a central figure in the 1930s political debate over malnutrition.[12]

Boyd Orr undertook his African tour in 1925 and predictably he reported that the main problem was that African grasslands were deficient in minerals. However, he concluded optimistically that the situation could be remedied by the use of fertilisers on the pastures and by dietary supplements for the livestock.[13] Towards the end of his time in Africa, Boyd Orr spent some time with the head of the Medical Department in Kenya, John Gilks. Together they undertook a survey of the diet and health of two African tribes, the Maasai and the Kikuyu, who lived adjacent to one another, but had very different cultures and very different dietary regimes. The Maasai lived mainly on meat and dairy products, whereas the Kikuyu diet was almost entirely a vegetarian one. The survey showed what was already suspected, namely that the Maasai had a better physique and enjoyed better health than the Kikuyu. Two issues emerged from the survey; firstly, the potential for comparative studies of the dietary determination of health and physique and secondly, the fact that the physique of Africans was poor, that they were susceptible to disease and that consequently labour was inefficient.[14]

Boyd Orr and Gilks' own initial findings appeared in the *Lancet* in March 1927.[15] The main emphasis in the article was on the poor nutritional status of the indigenous population of Africa and the fact that they suffered from a wide range of infectious and constitutional diseases. For Boyd Orr in particular the demonstration that the 'African native is . . . by no means the Noble Savage that he is frequently supposed to be', was ammunition against vegetarianism and the claims made for natural diets in the British debates on nutrition in the 1920s.[16] The main conclusion drawn was that greater attention, by the colonial authorities, to diet would increase the value of 'the native as an economic factor'.[17] At one level this survey was unremarkable in that all it did was to transfer to the colonies the kind of dietary surveys that were being carried out in Britain and elsewhere in the developed world. However, the way in which this happened and the fact that it happened at all was remarkable. Prior to this survey all matters of colonial health had been approached through the Colonial Medical Service and its own medical specialism, tropical medicine.[18] This specialism had been created and built up regarding the disease problems of the colonies as exclusively 'tropical' and thereby exotic; concentrating on vector-borne diseases like malaria and sleeping sickness, and on racial hygiene. Boyd Orr approached his work in East Africa with the universalist assumptions of a physiologically oriented nutritionist and without having been socialised into the exceptionalist assumptions of tropical medicine. Instead of seeing the usual differences between disease causation and occurrence in Europe and Africa he saw similarities. It was apparent that the metropolitan picture of tropical diseases was inaccurate. The main causes of death in East Africa were the world-wide scourges of pneumonia and tuberculosis. The commonest complaints were leg ulcers and dysentery and it was clear that 'cancer was by no means a rare disease'. The challenge to tropical medicine was not taken up and was in all probability not even seen. If it had been, the existing form of tropical medicine would have had to have been totally recast or perhaps it would have been rejected as a legitimate specialism.

Before all this was published, indeed immediately on his return from Africa and through his friend Walter Elliot, who was a member of the government, Boyd Orr discussed the significance of his work with Lord Balfour and Leopold Amery.[19] The result was a new CCR Sub-Committee on Dietetics, with a distinguished membership of Britain's leading nutritional scientists.[20] The brief of the Sub-Committee was to investigate dietetics in general not just in Africa, the belief was that the 'colonial laboratory' would provide excellent conditions for comparative nutritional research of imperial importance.[21] At the first meeting Boyd Orr submitted a programme of further investigations in Kenya involving chemical analysis of local foodstuffs, experiments with labour rations, a study of the aetiology of leg ulcers to explore malnutrition as a cause, and a full survey of the health and diet of the Maasai and the Kikuyu.[22] It was also announced that Gilks had already agreed to host the investigation and the Empire Marketing Board (EMB) was to provide a grant. All members of the Sub-Committee spoke enthusiastically about the proposal, although some were suspicious of Boyd Orr's objectivity with regard to the relative value of minerals as against vitamins. Two researchers were soon appointed and were in the field in the early months of 1927. Their work continued for four years and was published in 1931 by the Medical Research Council.[23]

The statistics on African mortality and morbidity given in the preliminary findings of Boyd Orr and Gilks in 1927 were restated and elaborated in the opening paragraphs of the Final Report in 1931, but the great bulk of the report concentrated on the new work on the dietary determination of health and physique. It was these latter findings that attracted most contemporary attention and which are cited to this day as one of the clearest demonstrations of dietary determinism. Indeed, their impact was particularly strong in anthropology where they stimulated research on the social and cultural influences and implications of diet.[24] It was argued, too, that the results showed the importance of a balanced diet, for although the Maasai were taller, heavier and healthier than the Kikuyu, they still showed certain patterns of disease that seemed to be linked to diet.[25] These findings contributed directly to British debates on nutritional research and food policy, which since the discovery of vitamins had emphasised specific deficiency diseases and their treatment by dietary supplements. That the report was received mainly as a contribution to dietetics obscured the fact that it also confirmed the earlier findings, 'that undernutrition, or malnutrition or more probably both, may occur to marked degree amongst native tribes'. Moreover the report concluded by suggesting that 'The problem is not confined to Kenya. It appears to exist in many different areas in our tropical dependencies. It may be judged . . . that the loss of health and efficiency attributable to deficient diet is, therefore, of considerable economic importance.'[26]

Although the final report recommended more research in both Africa and elsewhere, this work was not done. By the time the report was published in 1931, the CCR had been superceded by the less active and less interventionist Economic Advisory Council (EAC) and the EMB was about to be wound up.[27] Both changes resulted ultimately from the economic recession which hit medical and scientific research as hard as any area of government activity. In 1925, when the work had begun, there was much interest in the economic potential of East Africa and the Colonial Empire in general. After 1929 the outlook was less sanguine.[28] The Colonial Development Fund, established in that year, might seem to contradict this view, as it was presented as a means of stimulating economic activity in the colonies and increasing inter-imperial trade. However, it was at best a half-hearted measure and in reality it was more of a defensive measure designed to ameliorate the worst effects of the slump in Britain than to stimulate colonial development.[29] The British government, and for that matter British-based experts in nutrition and the medical sciences, seemed to forget about the issue of colonial nutrition until it was forced upon them again some years later by the work of the Health Division of the League of Nations.

Recognition

In 1933 the full Assembly of the League of Nations considered a *Report on Nutrition and Public Health.*[30] The Report brought together the results of the nutritional surveys that had been carried out in member countries in the previous decade and, on the strength of the evidence collected, argued that nutrition ought to be made an integral part of public health policy and administration. The claims made signalled the impending emergence of nutrition as a discipline in its own right and showed that a number of people were thinking about new professional opportunities for nutrition within public health. However, the professional identity and allegiance of 'nutritionists' was by no means clear for it was maintained that the subject was 'an economic, agricultural, industrial and commercial problem, as well as a problem of physiology'.[31] At an intellectual level nutrition was clearly interdisciplinary in character, embracing these and other fields. But at a practical and political level, it was so intricately bound up with economic concerns and political interests that the idea of disinterested professional expertise was always questionable. In the immediate future, however, it was assumed, wrongly as it turned out, that most workers in the field of nutrition would be linked to the biomedical science, medicine and public health.

The Third Volume of the League of Nations Report was devoted to what was identified as the 'new problem' of colonial dietary and the finding that 'it is now clear that colonial populations, in general, are undernourished'.[32] The implication throughout the document was that this situation had always existed due to backwardness and ignorance, but that this had recently been revealed by three changes. Firstly, of course, by the 'new knowledge' of nutrition and secondly, by the gradual extension of colonial medical services to the indigenous population.[33] Lastly, the Report made use of a number of surveys of the nutritional status of particular colonial populations, inspired by and modelled on that of Boyd Orr and Gilks, which had been carried out in other British and European colonies.[34] There is some validity in each of these explanations, but the number of surveys on which the League's Report made its claim about the generality and seriousness of colonial nutritional problems was not large. Also, it has to be remembered that what was being reported from the colonies was not malnutrition but undernutrition, and that the recognition of this was not dependent on the recent advance in nutrition.

There were other considerations that complicate any claim that there was a straightforward application of new knowledge to reveal a submerged, but perennial problem. Information on indigenous health and dietary had been available for many decades and had been compiled in vital statistics, labour reports, army recruitment data, annual medical reports, hospital records, medical missionary reports and earlier health surveys (e.g. on infant mortality). However, this data was not put to any systematic use until it was recovered and reused in the 'new' surveys of the 1930s. Indeed, it was exactly from sources of this kind that the Kenyan studies based their claims of the extent and seriousness of the overall nutritional problem in the colonies.[35] It is also worth noting that the 'colonial laboratory' had long been an important source of knowledge of deficiency diseases. The experiences of colonial medical personnel with various specialised and rationed diets had led to pioneering work being carried out, especially in the Far Eastern colonies (e.g. Eijkmann in the Dutch East Indies and Fletcher, Stanton and Fraser in the Federated Malay States all worked on beri-beri).[36] More well known is the work done in India on jail, barrack and famine relief diets, which culminated in the 1920s with the famous studies of Robert McCarrison.[37] In the 1930s Margaret Mellanby did pioneering research on the relation of diet and tooth decay in Kenya. Clearly, the flow of knowledge was not one way from centre to periphery, nor was it the case that 'pure' research was simply being applied to nutritional problems.

There was, in fact, a distinctive view of nutritional problems amongst colonial medical officers. Following the lead of McCarrison, they argued that too much attention was being given by European scientists to specific deficiency diseases and that the general effects of diet were being ignored. Colonial doctors were particularly interested in how a poor diet generally increased 'susceptibility to infection' and 'lowered vitality'.[38] Why this was so must, at this time, be a matter of speculation. It could be that it reflected their experiences of under-nutrition over and above the commoner European experience of mal-nutrition. As early as 1932, a joint conference of doctors from India and Africa had commented on the possible futility of colonial medical practice.

> In an undernourished population . . . the mere treatment of disease, no matter how effective and widely carried out, will achieve but negligible results. The first need is a continuous supply of sufficient and well-balanced food for the native to resist infection and the next is the improv-ment of housing. Both aspects depend on the economic status of the community.[39]

This meeting was one of the first of several inter-regional conferences that from the 1920s allowed members of the various colonial services to exchange experiences and perhaps develop a distinct collective view of colonial problems. Certainly the remoteness, both geographical and professional, of colonial medical officers from the growing influence of laboratory medicine in Europe may help to explain the persistence of a more holistic and hygienic conception of nutrition. In a recent paper, Smith and Nicolson have associated the similar anti-reductionist orientation of the Glasgow group of nutritionists (Paton, Finlay and Cathcart) with the conservative social values of a threatened elite[40]– in their particular case, clinicians who were threatened professionally by the rise of laboratory medicine and whose autonomy was threatened by wider political changes. Parallels with the position of colonial medical officers are not hard to find. The advances and new techniques of laboratory medicine had little relevance to colonial medical practice, especially to the work of district medical officers working 'up country'. The cutbacks in recruitment of the early 1930s would have exacerbated the situation, as the service became an aging one, trained in an earlier era of medicine. On top of this, the 1930s saw growing challenges to colonial rule, which included attacks on the technical services.

Uniquely, the British government saw the whole League of Nations Report not in terms of medicine or public health, but in the explicitly economic context of the world recession. Lord Astor, who became the chairman of the League's Committee on the Problem of Nutrition in 1935, summed up this view as follows:

> The marked interest which the last Assembly showed in nutrition was due, in the first instance, to the realisation of the possibility of great improvements in public health and social betterment through nutrition: but . . . the interest displayed was also due to the fact that through improved nutrition, it should be possible to contribute first towards a solution of national and international agricultural problems and secondly, towards an improvement in the world economic situation.[41]

At its simplest, increasing evidence of world hunger at a time of agricultural surpluses was seen as irrational. Thus, the League of Nations and scientistically-orientated groups and individuals sought to plan a new world agricultural order. The League's report in 1937 on *The Relation of Health, Agriculture and Economic Policy*, the *World Food Plan* of 1938, and the United Nations Food and Agriculture Organisation formed in 1944 were all outcomes of this interest.[42] As far as the administration of the British Colonial Empire was concerned the effects of the recession were more complex. It has already been suggested that the government attempted to use the colonies to soften the impact of the depression by initiating proposals to bind the Empire economies closer to Britain – for example, the Colonial Development Fund and imperial preference in 1932. At the same time, since the colonies as primary producers were very hard hit by the fall in commodity prices and the consequent loss of income, they were not well placed to bale Britain out. While there was much talk of 'development', the reality was that in most colonies there was economic stagnation and even a withdrawal into subsistence.[43] These economic difficulties, together with political unrest and the nascent independence movements they fostered, meant that the problems of the colonies were too pressing to be ignored. Furthermore, the government had to face the criticism of a growing number of intellectuals who argued that imperial responsibilities were not only being overlooked, but were not even understood.[44] These concerns were exemplified by the new paternalism of initiatives like Lord Hailey's 'African Survey' and the complementary scientific survey undertaken by E. B. Worthington.[45]

Thus, while impelled to action by the League of Nations, when the

British government officially took up the matter of nutrition in the colonies it defined the issue structurally, as one of agricultural and economic development, rather than of medical services and public health. A circular issued in 1936 announced that a major survey of colonial malnutrition would be organised by a sub-committee of the EAC.[46] The circular asked colonial governments, firstly, to provide information on the nutritional status of their indigenous populations and, secondly, to explore agricultural policies with a view to achieving a better balance between export crops and domestic food crops, as 'increased attention to dietetic need might well lead to an amelioration of . . . economic problems'.[47]

Solutions

The EAC Committee on Nutrition in the Colonial Empire met on only four occasions between its formation in 1936 and the publication of its final report in 1939. The scientific aspects of the problem were devolved to an expert Research Sub-Committee, while the collation of responses to the 1936 circular and the drafting of the report was left to the Committee Secretaries.[48] The work of the Research Sub-Committee endorsed the earlier conclusions that there was no fundamental difference between the physiology of the tropical races and that of Europeans and argued that field surveys rather than laboratory research was now required. They advised that it was a waste of time stipulating an 'ideal diet' because the average diet in tropical countries, under present conditions, 'falls so far short of the ideal'.[49] More and more evidence to support such a view was being received month by month by the main Committee as replies to the Secretary of State's circular came in.

Each colony responded to the request for information in a different way. Most commonly, reports were written by the director of the medical service or the agricultural service, although in a number of cases reports were drawn up by local legislative bodies or specially constituted local nutrition committees. In a few colonies new field surveys were undertaken, but, in the main, existing documentation and the 'experience' of local officials was relied upon. In Trinidad, for example, the Governor appointed a representative group and their report drew on local vital statistics, a limited new dietary survey, medical reports and economic intelligence.[50] A large part of the evidence collected pointed to ignorance of dietetics amongst the native population and the fact that native diets were badly balanced. However, there was no escaping the conclusion that the problem went beyond dietetics.

> The [EAC] Committee will also have to face the problem of underfeeding which is usually due to poverty, but sometimes is the result of ignorance. Poverty is fundamentally an economic question which lies beyond the scope of our Committee to handle.[51]

The same point was made by the Governor of Antigua who wrote, quoting his Senior Medical Officer, that 'The chief factor in Antigua is the economic . . . I have investigated numerous cases of malnutrition in infants and in practically every case poverty is the cause. Parents cannot afford to buy food.'[52] Identical messages came from West Africa and the Far East. Reports from West Africa pointed to evidence of a deterioration in native health since the nineteenth century; in the case of Sierra Leone this was linked directly to 'lack of husbandry' and worsening dietary.[53] The Director of the Medical Department in the Gold Coast seemed to make a direct connection with the consequences of an export-oriented colonial economy.

> So much attention has been devoted to the cocoa and mining industries that the fact that the majority of inhabitants are simple village farmers living chiefly on food produced on their farms is apt to be overlooked. The need, therefore, to conserve forests and to improve on the present wasteful system of shifting cultivation by the education of farmers in the intensive methods and in the relative food values of his crops is one which cannot but strike the observer.[54]

From Mauritius came the statement that:

> There is an impression prevalent among many employers that the field labourers of today are decidedly less robust than those of a generation or more ago and that tasks performed are smaller. This impression is supported by the opinion of the Protector of Immigrants and the Poor Law Commissioner.[55]

Only from East Africa did replies suggest the main problem was malnutrition rather than undernutrition, no doubt reflecting the findings of the Boyd Orr surveys.[56] The only other report that stood out was that from Ceylon, where overpopulation and the long-standing backwardness of colonial peoples were thought to be the major cause of nutritional problems.[57] But the great bulk of evidence from all the other colonies did suggest that serious nutritional problems were of recent origin. The common perception was that the people's health had deteriorated in recent times.

On the basis of the evidence accumulated over eighteen months, a Draft Report was prepared by the Secretaries and circulated in March 1938.[58] In the main the draft faithfully followed the conclusions of the local reports and identified poverty and then ignorance as the main causes of malnutrition in the colonies. Poverty was seen to be produced by inadequate production of food crops, low wages and poor yields, and by colonies receiving insufficient returns for their export crops. Ignorance was attributed not to the native population but to 'Government officials and those who have power over the nutrition of others, e.g. employers, missionaries and teachers'.[59] In one sense this report could be read as an indictment of colonial policy and of colonialism itself. Certainly its analysis was congruent with what Hetherington has defined as 'the Colonial Problem':

> [This] was concerned with the general problems of development, with an attempt to provide some sort of guide to solutions. [It] emphasised that the interests of the native population were primary, and dealt with such problems as the building up of internal capital, the prevention of undue drainage of wealth from the colonies, and problems associated with a proper balance between agricultural production for home consumption and for export.[60]

Criticisms of colonial policy, even from official bodies, were not uncommon in the late thirties. For example, the findings of the West India Royal Commission were so controversial that its publication was delayed from 1939 until 1945.[61] The views of many African scholars were summed up by Audrey Richards in 1939, when she wrote that the diet and health of colonial peoples 'has deteriorated in contact with white civilisation rather than the reverse'.[62] For her, at least, colonial malnutrition was a modern epidemic.

The Draft Report should be read, however, less as a critique of colonialism *per se* and more as an acknowledgement that colonial policies were not working as well as they should and might even be self-defeating. Most local reports pointed to the particularly severe effects of the world recession on the colonies and their peoples. Local revenue was hit as trade slumped, retrenchment was forced on colonial companies and the colonial service, including the medical service, was cut back. In the Draft Report, the indigenous population was seen as being entirely passive; it was given no role in improving conditions and by implication it seems to be argued that nutritional problems were not of their making. It was suggested that even 'ignorance' was something the colonial authorities should have tackled. The problem of colonial malnutrition was constructed as one of colonial agencies requiring new policies and programmes. Existing policies were said to have been ill-informed, ineffective and counterproductive. Comments of this kind echoed fears that colonial agricultural experts had been expressing about the economic and ecological consequences of monoculture and shifting cultivation. Indeed, between the wars, the colonial science of tropical agriculture changed from being a crop-based, plantation-orientated discipline, to one concerned with wider agricultural systems, embracing food as well as cash crops.[63] The favoured policy amongst colonial agriculturalists, again showing the breakdown of tropical exceptionalism, was to introduce into the colonies the then fashionable British practices of 'mixed farming' and 'green manuring'.[64] It was, in fact, mainly colonial agriculturalists who linked malnutrition and population growth, but even then population growth was an emerging trend rather than a cause of existing problems.[65] Also, they always linked population growth and soil erosion, to produce an analysis whereby any future improvement of colonial agriculture would be threatened by both supply (loss of land) and demand (growth of population).

Most members of the main Committee accepted the Draft Report. However, the response of one member, Professor N. F. Hall, led to a major rewriting and reorganisation of the document.[66] Hall objected to the emphasis the document gave to the low economic level of the colonies and argued that food crops should be developed at the expense of cash crops and other exports. He claimed that any moves that could be seen as making colonial produce more expensive or less accessible or both would be 'politically dynamite'.[67] He suggested that the whole Report should instead give far more attention to dietetic and nutritional matters. 'The state of knowledge with regard to the economic issues involved is, I think, considerably less than that with regard to the beneficial properties of certain types of foodstuffs.'[68] An incidental and no doubt intended consequence of this change of emphasis was to shift the tone of the Report from one of pessimism to one of optimism. The emphasis on intractable, structural problems gave way to the notion that the problems were soluble by known, practical measures that the government could introduce.

It took over a year to rewrite the Report and the changes made were substantial.[69] The main argument was still that the low standard of living and ignorance were at the root of the problem, but the former point was not made as strongly as it had been before. The causes were now discussed in a rather academic way in a section headed 'The General Character of the Problem' rather than the more direct, original section on 'The Causes of Malnutition and Practical Measures to Relieve It'.[70] More generally, the Final Report was fill out out with large, new sections on nutritional topics such as, 'Desirable Additions to Colonial Diets', 'The Harvesting, Preservation, Storage, Processing and Cooking of Foods' and 'The Purchase of Foodstuffs'. The Committee certainly received advice on optimal diets from the Ministry of

Health's Advisory Committee on Nutrition and this was ultimately recommended to the colonies, in spite of the fact that its own expert Research Sub-Committee had said such standards were irrelevant.

In both versions colonial malnutrition was defined primarily as an agricultural problem. In the first draft this was presented as a matter of political economy; in the second version it was a matter of 'native education'. The 'native' was pictured here as being caught in a vicious circle of ignorance, poverty and disease. Disease was being tackled by the medical services, poverty was dependent on world economic forces, so that left ignorance as the only area where worthwhile recommendations could be made. As the analysis of the Report unfolded, it was increasingly contended that ignorance was the root cause of poverty and disease, and the point where the vicious circle could be most effectively broken. If people knew what to grow, how to grow it, what to eat and how to cook it, then there would be less poverty and hence less disease. Who would direct the 'ignorant natives' in good agricultural and dietetic practice? Why the very same colonial agencies that the Draft Report had condemned for their ignorance! Overall, the problem of colonial malnutrition had become one that was seen to be soluble by the deployment of appropriate expertise and co-operation between nutritional experts, agriculturalists, doctors, anthropologists, teachers and economists. In short, nutrition had been transformed from being conceptualised as a major structural problem to being conceptualised as a technical problem.

Conclusion

When the report on Nutrition in the Colonial Empire was finally published in July 1939, it attracted very little professional, public or political attention.[71] This was only partly a result of its conclusions having been emasculated during drafting. By that time the Report was saying nothing new, for after 1936 the problem of nutrition in the Colonial Empire had been widely debated in colonial circles, and in medical and agricultural journals.[72] However, the main reason for its being ignored was almost certainly the unfolding political crisis in Europe and the view that any question of colonial development would now have to await the outcome of the impending conflict.

In the Report evidence can be found to support each of the three main explanations of the origins of malnutrition in developing countries. This is not surprising, as it would be unlikely that any single explanation would cover the diversity of cultures and economic systems found in the Colonial Empire. One significant aspect of the

Report, and this is true of colonial policy on agricultural, medical and scientific matters too, is that the diversity of the colonies was obscured by the assumption that all colonies had a common tropical environment and uniformly backward peoples. An administrative entity became a 'natural' entity. The weight of evidence in the Report does point, not only to the problem of colonial malnutrition only being conceptualised in the 1930s, but to the fact that it was a new phenomenon on the ground in the colonies. Interestingly, in the light of more recent discussion, population growth was hardly mentioned as a significant factor. The explanations of the problem given are the effects of the world recession, the disruption of traditional agricultural practices, the application of new nutritional knowledge and the new attitudes to colonial peoples.

The 'discovery' of colonial malnutrition was a result of the direct transfer of the 'dietary survey' from the centre to the periphery. The important point was that the transfer was direct and did not involve the creation of an exceptionalist, tropical nutritional science. Rooted in the basic sciences of physiology and biochemistry, nutritional science allowed a common approach to problems worldwide, which subjects like tropical medicine and tropical agriculture had previously denied. The emerging experts in nutrition and those who applied their techniques were, therefore, the key agency in revealing the new disease picture of the colonies. The subsequent 'recognition' of malnutrition by colonial policy-makers was almost entirely dependent on the effects of the world recession on world agriculture and colonial economies. Indigenous populations were naively seen as a potential market for world agricultural surpluses and more immediately the growing political pressure on the imperial powers both from within and from without meant that such problems had to be confronted or at least seen to be confronted. As always, the official response of calling an investigation looked constructive and could always be held out as the precursor to effective action. The characterisation of the problem before 1938 was undoubtedly that it was primarily economic and this was clearly linked with wider reactions against colonialism. The association of nutritional survey work with radical political views was not uncommon in Britain in the 1930s. But as in Britain, the technical dimensions of the problem allowed for this radicalism to be lost as the definition of the problem changed from one of inappropriate structures to one of inadequate knowledge. The eventual stress that was put on native 'ignorance' and the general backwardness of the colonies allowed evidence of the recent origins of the problem to be ignored. Colonial malnutrition was rapidly and readily reconstructed from being seen as an epidemic problem to an endemic one, for which colonialism had little responsibility and over which it could exercise little control.

Notes

This chapter is based on work supported by an award from the SRC/SSRC, undertaken during the preparation of my D.Phil. dissertation. A version of this chapter was given as a paper at the Annual Conference of the Society for the Social History of Medicine in Sheffield in 1986. A summary appeared in the *Bulletin of the Society for the Social History of Medicine,* XL, 1987. I would like to thank David Arnold for his helpful comments on an earlier draft. This final version is, of course, entirely my responsibility.

1 E. V. McCollum, *A History of Nutrition: A Sequence of Ideas in Nutritional Investigations,* Boston, Mass., 1957, p. 421. A recent review reveals the paucity of historical studies in this area, see D. Grigg, *The World Food Problem, 1950–1980,* Oxford, 1985. Cf. P. D. Curtin, 'Nutrition in African history', *Journal of Interdisciplinary History,* XIV, 1983, pp. 371-82.

2 For example, see R. Dumont and B. Rosier, *The Hungry Future,* London, 1969. Cf. S. George, *How the Other Half Dies: The Real Reasons for World Hunger,* Harmondsworth, 1977.

3 J. de Castro, *The Geography of Hunger,* London, 1965; W. Rodney, *How Europe Underdeveloped Africa,* London, 1972.

4 For an exception see R. Maulitz, 'Channel crossing: the lure of French pathology for English medical students, 1816–1836', *Bulletin of the History of Medicine,* LV, 1982, pp. 475–96.

5 G. Lemaine et al (eds.), *The Emergence of New Scientific Disciplines,* Paris, 1976.

6 J. Habermas, *Towards a Rational Society,* London, 1971; P. Conrad and J. W. Schneider (eds.), *Deviance and Medicalisation: From Badness to Sickness,* St Louis, 1980.

7 C. Petty, 'Food, poverty and growth: the application of nutrition science, 1918–1939', *Bulletin of the Society for the Social History of Medicine,* XL, 1987.

8 R. MacLeod and E. K. Andrews, 'The Committee of Civil Research: scientific advice for economic development, 1925–1930', *Minerva,* IV, 1969, pp. 680-705. The papers of the Committee on the Mineral Content of Pastures are in the Cabinet Papers at the Public Record Office, Kew, London, CAB 58/96 CR(MC) and CAB 58/109 CR(D).

9 CAB 58/96 CR(C)6.

10 *Biographical Memoirs of Fellows of the Royal Society,* XVIII, 1972, pp. 43-81 and Lord Boyd Orr, *As I Recall,* London, 1966.

11 H. Melville, *The D.S.I.R.,* London, 1962; A. Landsborough Thomson, *Half A Century of Medical Research,* II, London, 1973, pp. 73-90.

12 Boyd Orr, *As I Recall, passim.*

13 CAB 58/96 CR(MC)14, Report dated 10 March 1926.

14 CAB 58/109 CR(D)1 and 2.

15 J. L. Gilks and J. B. Orr, 'The nutritional condition of the East African Native', *The Lancet,* i, 1927, pp. 561-2.

16 *Ibid.,* p. 562.

17 *Ibid.,* p. 561.

18 M. Worboys, *Science and British Colonial Imperialism, 1895–1940,* unpublished D.Phil. thesis, University of Sussex, 1980, pp. 83-141.

19 At this time the development of the Empire was attracting the attention of leading politicians such as Lord Balfour, Leopold Amery and William Ormsby-Gore. Also it was particularly associated with science, on this see Worboys, *Science,* pp. 214-21. Walter Elliot, who can be seen as a member of the 'science for development group' completed a doctorate at Rowett on animal nutrition while a government minister.

20 The Sub-Committee were Walter Elliot (chair), Sir Frederick Hopkins, Professor E. P. Cathcart, Sir Walter Fletcher, Dr J. B. Orr and Dr G. J. Rutherford.

21 CAB 58/96 CR(C)16 23 July 1926.

22 *Ibid.*
23 J. Boyd Orr and J. L. Gilks, *Studies in Nutrition: The Physique and Health of Two African Tribes*, London, 1931.
24 A. I. Richards, *Hunger and Work in a Savage Tribe*, London, 1932; R. Firth, 'The sociological study of native diet', *Africa*, VII, 1934, pp. 401-14.
25 Boyd Orr, *Studies*, p. 46.
26 *Ibid.*, p. 49.
27 Worboys, *Science*, pp. 272-80.
28 *Ibid.*, p. 244-94.
29 E. A. Brett, *Colonialism and Underdevelopment in East Africa: The Politics of Economic Change, 1919–1939*, London, 1973.
30 E. Burnet and W. R. Aykroyd, 'Nutrition and public health', *Quarterly Bulletin of the Health Organisation of the League of Nations*, IV, June 1935, pp. 1-140.
31 *Ibid.*, p. 1.
32 *Ibid.*, p. 126.
33 C. Jeffries, *The Colonial Empire and its Civil Service*, London, 1938, Appendix; A. Beck, *A History of the British Medical Administration of East Africa, 1900–1950*, Cambridge, Mass., 1970.
34 For example, W. E. McCulloch, 'An inquiry into the dietaries of the Hausas and Town Fulani of Northern Nigeria', *West African Medical Journal*, III, 1929–30; G. Hardy and C. Richet, *L'Alimentation indigène dans les Colonies Français*, Paris, 1932.
35 Boyd Orr, *Studies*, pp. 17-19.
36 C. Singer and E. A. Underwood, *A Short History of Medicine*, Oxford, 1962, pp. 610–2.
37 R. McCarrison, *Studies in Deficiency Diseases*, Oxford, 1921.
38 CAB 58/109 EAC(D)12 and EAC(D)16.
39 'Report on an International Conference of representatives of health services of African Territories and British India', *Quarterly Bulletin of the Health Organisation of the League of Nations*, II, 1933, p. 115.
40 D. Smith and M. Nicolson, 'Paton, Cathcart and Findlay: a conservative stance in Scottish nutrition', *Bulletin of the Society for the Social History of Medicine*, XL, 1987.
41 *The Problem of World Nutrition*, I, Geneva, 1936, p. 5.
42 *Final Report of the Mixed Committee of the League of Nations on the Relation of Nutrition to Health, Agriculture and Economic Policy*, Geneva, 1937. An outline of activities to remedy the 'world food problem' at this time is given in J. Boyd Orr and D. Lubbock, *The White Man's Dilemma*, London, 1965, pp. 49-58.
43 A. G. Hopkins, *An Economic History of West Africa*, London, 1973, pp. 254-66.
44 P. Hetherington, *British Paternalism and Africa, 1920–1940*, London, 1978, *passim*.
45 Lord Hailey, *An African Survey*, London, 1938; E. B. Worthington, *Science in Africa*, London, 1938.
46 *Nutritional Policy in the Colonial Empire*, Colonial 121, London, 1936, para. 3; and CAB 58/199 EAC (NCE)1.
47 *Nutritional Policy in the Colonial Empire*, para. 8.
48 The membership of the Research Sub-Committee was Sir Edward Mellanby, Professor E. P. Cathcart, Sir J. Boyd Orr, Sir T. Stanton and Dr A. I Richards. The main Committee met on only four occasions: 21 November 1936, 24 March 1937, 1 December 1937 and 3 April 1939. The Committee Secretaries were two Colonial Office civil servants D. H. F. Ricketts and C. G. Eastwood.
49 CAB 58/199 EAC(NCE)(R)8, p. 16.
50 CAB 58/208 EAC(NCE)26, Report of the Nutrition Committee, Trinidad, 1936. All of the information received by the Committee was published in summary form in *Nutrition in the Colonial Empire, Report of the Economic Advisory Council.* part I, PP, 1938-39, [Cmd. 6050], X, p. 265.
51 *Ibid.*, no pagination in the report from Trinidad.
52 CAB 58/199 EAC(NCE)45.
53 CAB 58/199 EAC(NCE)65.

54 CAB 58/199 EAC(NCE)35. Quoted from the Annual Report of the Medical Department, 1934, p. 7.
55 CAB 58/199 EAC(NCE)40.
56 CAB 58/199 EAC(NCE)63.
57 CAB 58/199 EAC(NCE)45, Report on Nutrition in Ceylon, Sessional Paper II, 1937, p. 11.
58 CAB 58/208 EAC(NCE)(D)5.
59 *Ibid.*
60 Hetherington, *British Paternalism*, p. 100.
61 *Recommendations of the West India Royal Commission*, PP, 1939–40, [Cmd. 6174], v, p. 245.
62 A. I. Richards, *Land, Labour and Diet in North Rhodesia: An Economic Study of the Bemba Tribe*, London, 1939, p. 1. On Audrey Richards's work see J. Gladstone, '"Venturing on the Borderline": Audrey Richards's ethnographic contribution to the "Hungry Thirties" debate in Africa, 1927–1942', *Bulletin of the Society for the Social History of Medicine*, XL, 1987; J. Gladstone, 'Significant sister: autonomy and obligation in Audrey Richards' early fieldwork', *American Ethnologist*, XIII, 1986, pp. 338–61.
63 G. B. Masefield, *A History of the Colonial Agricultural Service*, London, 1972.
64 O. T. Faulkner and J. R. Mackie, *West African Agriculture*, London, 1933; and G. R. Morrison, *Mixed Farming in East Africa*, London, 1935.
65 D. Hall, *The Improvement of Native Agriculture in Relation to Population and Public Health*, London, 1936.
66 CAB 58/206 EAC(NCE)(D)7. Professor Hall held the Chair of Political Economy at the University of London. He was not a particularly well known or influential economist, so it is likely his comments were supported by others within the EAC and the Colonial Office.
67 *Ibid.*
68 *Ibid.*
69 CAB 58/208 EAC(NCE)(D)5; and *Nutrition in the Colonial Empire, Report of the Economic Advisory Council*, part 1, PP, 1938–39, (Cmd. 6051), X, p. 55.
70 *Nutrition*, part I, paras. 90-3.
71 'Nutrition in the Colonial Empire', *British Medical Journal*, ii, (1939), pp. 294-6; 'Nutrition in the Colonies', *The Times*, 26 July 1939, p. 15; and Lord Hailey, 'The native and his diet: malnutrition in the Colonies', *The Times*, 28 July 1939, pp. 15-16.
72 In April 1936 the journal *Africa* had published a special issue on the subject of the African native diet.

INDEX

INDEX

INDEX

INDEX